THE
CONSCIOUS I

W9-DDQ-346

THE CONSCIOUS I

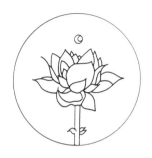

CLARITY AND DIRECTION THROUGH MEDITATION

A Handbook for Radical Change

ANDY JAMES

A PATRICK CREAN BOOK

SOMERVILLE HOUSE PUBLISHING,
Toronto

Copyright © 1992 by Andy James

All rights reserved. No part of this publication may be
reproduced or transmitted in any form or by any means —
electronic or mechanical, including photocopy, recording or any
information storage and retrieval system — without written
permission from the Publisher, except by a reviewer who wishes
to quote brief passages for inclusion in a review.

CANADIAN CATALOGUING IN PUBLICATION DATA

James, Andy, 1949–
The conscious I : clarity and direction through meditation

ISBN 0-921051-76-X

1. Meditation. 2. Meditation — Buddhism.
3. Stress (Psychology). I. Title.

BQ5572.J36 1992   294.3'444   C92-094540-6

Cover and text design: Tania Craan
Cover Art: Marcia Masino
Printed in Canada

A PATRICK CREAN BOOK

Published by Somerville House Publishing,
a division of Somerville House Books Limited,
3080 Yonge Street, Suite 5000, Toronto, Ontario M4N 3N1

Somerville House Publishing acknowledges the
financial assistance of the Ontario Arts Council.

I dedicate this book to my Vipassana teacher, Dhiravamsa, to my wife, Yolind, to my children — Shu Wen, Shu Wei, Hana — and to my students. All have helped me along the path of Insight and Compassion.

I am deeply grateful to Ann Wee for her long-standing support and encouragement.

CONTENTS

INTRODUCTION

I think of my life as ordinary, and I feel great about it. Yet something extraordinary must have happened to make me give up the status and financial security of a sober profession (I was a chartered accountant) for the precariousness and, at times, ridicule of life as a teacher of meditation and Tai Chi. In 1984, when I made that leap into the unknown, I also had a wife and two young children to support.

The nearest thing to a "Eureka!" experience in my life was reading Christmas Humphreys' *Buddhism*. I read it not out of any interest in Buddhism but to amass anti-religious ammunition for my arguments with the trendy proponents of Zen. It was the end of the sixties, and the student revolutionary movement was in full swing; I was in England studying at the London School of Economics and Political Science, long-famous as a breeding ground for political and social activists.

One aspect of Buddhism really struck me. While as a faith it was faultlessly logical, it regarded the intellect as limited, incapable of providing all the answers. Moreover, unlike other religions I had encountered, it did not demand belief; it did not lay claim to an exclusive revelation from God. The Buddha was not God but a human being who had found complete enlightenment. His message was that each person could do the same, by looking inward.

Buddhism invites careful inspection of all phenomena, external as well as internal. Instead of refining the *contents* of your belief systems, you are encouraged to go deeper and look at the *process* of belief. It is a challenge to the intellect (and therefore to one's own sense of "self" or "I") to enquire into the mechanisms of its own limitations and insecurities. Usually we want to get rid of our problems; we do not like to acknowledge the possibility that we ourselves might be the problem.

I had always accepted society's view of the intellect as omnipotent and the sole legitimate source of good judgement. The sudden realization that it was not omnipotent clarified many long-standing puzzles for me: why humanity's endless attempts at Utopia fail (and are immediately replaced by new versions), why the revolutionaries always become the new establishment, and why we do not learn from history or from our life experiences nearly as much as we think we do.

I was elated to discover that life need not be just a series of dead-end tunnels. There was indeed light in the tunnel, and amazingly the source of that light was within myself. My life since that moment has been an irresistible and always surprising exploration of that light. The more I journeyed inward, the clearer life's meaning became and the more connected I felt with my environment.

Although Humphreys' book on Buddhism was the spark for these realizations, I had been primed by three occurrences.

The first was my discovery of the martial arts. For the first time in my life, I was able to give myself to something totally. The martial arts seemed real and honest — no "civilized" rules or equipment to mask the primordial confrontation of one person against another. There was no place to run, no rationalizations to be made. Size and brute strength were not the only weapons; speed, agility, bravery and intelligence could be even more powerful. I loved the martial arts, and discovered that I had a talent for them.

The martial arts not only initiated a process of mind-body exploration but also reconnected me to my Oriental heritage. They led me to the practice of Hatha Yoga and, eventually, to Chinese philosophy and history. I had grown up in the tiny colony of British Guiana, the only English-speaking country in South America, where the Chinese constituted only one-half percent of the population. The predominant cultural influences were British and American. Although my family was Anglican, I went to a Roman Catholic primary school, where the Jesuits thought I had great potential to join their order. I had never heard of Taoism, and I knew Confucianism only in the context of jokes or fortune cookies: "Confucius say . . ."

My second "primer" was a car crash in the Norwegian mountains in the summer of 1969. I was literally inches away from plunging off a cliff into the fjord below. After the accident, I spent a seemingly endless weekend in a tiny village with nothing to do but sit in my room and contemplate my fragile mortality — quite a disturbing experience for a twenty-year-old. It was my first spontaneous meditation, and afterwards I felt a strong need to deepen this type of inner examination.

The third significant event around the same time was meeting Yolind, who would become my wife. Her father (a distant second cousin of mine from Singapore) was Chinese and her mother was English, which in many ways made her like me — Chinese, yet not. She helped me to further explore my Chinese heritage, especially during our annual visits to Singapore. As with the martial arts, she enabled me to give of myself without holding back. For the first time in a relationship, I did not need to be in control. I discovered love . . . and the pain of vulnerability.

The elation resulting from my discovery of Buddhism was tinged with fear and the sense of loss. Although its truth was undeniable to me, I knew that if I pursued Buddhism my life would change drastically, which at that point I did not want. I could not, however, stop myself from exploring this new universe that had been revealed to me. I read voraciously about Buddhism, Taoism, Eastern and Western mysticism, Hinduism, Zen, comparative religion and the occult. I experimented with various forms of meditation and mind control.

As I continued my practices, many old habits and patterns simply began to fall away without much conscious effort. This was sometimes painful, especially if it involved other people, but it was not a matter of choice; what needed to be done was so obvious as to be beyond choosing. It became crystal clear to me that there was no "easy way" to live, no successful strategy for circumventing the law of cause and effect. What needs doing is best done now.

The year 1974 was one of significant beginnings. It was the start of my life as a fully qualified chartered accountant, but at a deeper level it was also the end, because that was the year I found my two main esoteric teachers.

I met my Insight Meditation teacher, Dhiravamsa, when I decided to intensify my meditation practice and join a formal group. I had been attracted to Insight Meditation, or Vipassana, years earlier, but had wanted to "play the field" and had tried various forms of meditation. Eventually I came back to Insight Meditation because of its simplicity and its profundity. Its goal is not peace, bliss or "spiritual" feeling but clarity and total action in each moment. It seemed to me that if one could achieve that, nothing else would be necessary.

Dhiravamsa was an impressive enigma. He emanated the deep inner clarity and power that one might expect of someone who had lived the monastic life for twenty-three years and who had occupied a senior position in the Thai Buddhist hierarchy. Yet here he was in the comfortable English countryside, open, accessible and "ordinary," with no hint of spiritual superiority. Although he was one of the first recognized Buddhist meditation masters to come to the West, he had given up his status within the Buddhist community to pioneer, within the context of traditional Buddhist meditation, the use of techniques from other spiritual disciplines and from psychotherapy. Today, more than twenty years later, the value of such an approach is widely recognized; back then, he was considered a black sheep.

For me, the interaction with other people, which Dhiravamsa's approach entailed, was much more difficult than solitary sitting meditation. (For others, it might be the other way around.) My early retreats with Dhiravamsa were arduous and intense, but immensely purifying. A few weeks of meditation retreat seemed the equivalent of years of "real time" living and learning. The wisdom/insight aspect of the practice was easy for me. My lesson seemed to be about opening the heart: giving, trusting, loving, allowing myself to be vulnerable and to experience pain, allowing life to reveal its surprises.

My other important mentor was a Tai Chi Chuan teacher, Rose Li. She was the only surviving daughter of a Beijing Mandarin family that had known more prosperous times. At the age of eight, she was slowly dying despite both Chinese and Western medical treatment. As a last resort, she was referred to a famous Beijing master of the Chinese internal martial arts — Tai Chi Chuan, Ba Gua and Hsing Yi — and she regained her health. She felt she owed her life to her teacher and to these martial arts. She regarded it as her duty not only to share her knowledge of them but to preserve their integrity. Teaching to her was like passing on a family heirloom.

Rose Li was studying in the United States when the Revolution broke out in China, marooning her in the West. Like Dhiravamsa, she was one of the first genuine teachers in her field in the West. I was fortunate to study with her soon after she emigrated to England to escape the melting pot of American culture.

Although I found Tai Chi slow at first, it has proven to be a major force in my life. Not only is it a sophisticated and powerful martial art and mind-body exercise, but a moving meditation that wholly complements the practice of Insight Meditation. I see Tai Chi Chuan in essence as balance between yin and yang in all its innumerable forms — inner and outer, movement and stillness, man and woman, advancing and retreating, softness and hardness.

Yolind and I were married in 1975, following this year of significant beginnings. In 1981, expecting our first child and feeling somewhat stagnant in England, we immigrated to Canada. I worked in Toronto for two years as an accountant in my family's business, but each day it became more difficult for me to perform my tasks. For years my heart had been drifting away from accountancy, even though my intellect kept insisting that it was the reasonable thing to do since it assured financial security for my growing family.

During a 1983 retreat at Dhiravamsa's meditation centre on San Juan Island off the coast of Washington, my teacher invited me to come live with him and be trained as a meditation teacher. My first reaction was to brush this invitation aside as preposterously impractical, since we were now a family of three (shortly to be four); we had no savings to finance such an adventure and the prospects of earning a living as a meditation teacher were extremely dim. A few minutes later, however, I agreed.

During the year my family and I lived on San Juan Island, I grew very close to Dhiravamsa, valuing him not only as an open, accessible and enlightened teacher but as a loving friend. I also found the courage to keep on trusting and following my "heart" — not my whims or fantasies — no matter how improbable and insecure this might have seemed. I completed the manuscript of my first book and decided to return to Toronto to undertake the highly unpromising task of establishing myself as a teacher of Insight Meditation and Tai Chi Chuan.

Following the light has not been easy. Financial insecurity and having such different ideas compared to most other people have at times placed a great strain on my marriage. On the other hand, life now makes much more sense and is more real, more intense and fuller, I hope, for my family and students as well as for myself. It continues to be a fascinating and unpredictable journey, with the next step always the greatest challenge. As I look back on my life at the age of forty-three, I feel no pain, no regrets. In spite of my commitments to my family, students and friends, I feel free.

I have written this book to share some of the teachings, insights and experiences that have helped me, my loved ones and my students make radical changes in our lives.

Radical change is necessary not only for our personal health and fulfilment but also, I am sure, for our survival as a species. What we see in the world around us is the result not of bad luck but of a lack of self-knowledge. Most of us mean well and see the necessity for urgent change but keep on doing things in fundamentally the same way we always have, albeit with different tools and rationales.

The clarity and direction necessary for achieving real change is within our reach right now. Few attain this inner wisdom because it threatens our present world view. Insight is not a thing to be grasped, but a way of living. If you learn that way, you can achieve a direct understanding of matters that may take years or decades of scientific research to substantiate. You simply know and act in accordance with that knowing. Such action is total and harmonious, clear and compassionate.

I hope this book will explain why real change is so elusive and what each of us can do to bring it about.

I

THE CHALLENGE
OF CHANGE

"Manage the difficult while they are easy;
Manage the great while they are small.

. . .

All difficult things in the world start from the easy;
All great things in the world start from the small.

. . .

A thousand miles' journey begins from the spot under one's feet.

. . .

The sage never attempts great things and thus can achieve
what is great."
— *LAO-TZU*, THE TAO TE CHING

"We must never relax our efforts to arouse in the people of
the world, and especially in their governments, an awareness
of the unprecedented disaster which they are absolutely cer-
tain to bring on themselves unless there is a fundamental
change in their attitudes toward one another as well as in
their concept of the future. The unleashed power of the atom
has changed everything save our modes of thinking."*
— *ALBERT EINSTEIN*

*I chose this quotation before the collapse of the Soviet Union but I have let it stand because the threat of nuclear destruction, although now on a smaller scale, is still very real. Einstein's observation applies to all forms of power, not just atomic: greater power necessitates greater spiritual maturity and wisdom.

The clamour for urgent, radical change is ringing from all corners of our planet with mounting frequency and intensity. Whether the issue is world peace, Third World or local poverty, violence against women and children, militant fundamentalism, AIDS, or the drug epidemic and its associated ills, there is a sense of crisis, a feeling that we need to do something before the quality of life deteriorates beyond the point of no return. The planet is ailing and is being pushed towards the limits of its recuperative powers. We are disoriented by the rapid and profound changes taking place all around us. As the pace of life quickens, the old rules become obsolete faster. We are forced to make up new rules as we go along without having understood why the old ones failed us. As a result, most of us experience confusion and persistent stress in our lives; life feels like a struggle.

Stress and Adapting to Change

It is no coincidence that *stress* is a major watchword of our time. It is the direct result of our failure to adapt to our rapidly changing environment. Rather than change our way of thinking (that is, adapt inwardly) as Einstein suggested, most of us still turn for relief to the very technology that created many of the stressors in the first place.

Stress has a formal name, the General Adaptation Syndrome. Dr. Hans Selye, its "discoverer" and one of the world's foremost authorities on stress, described this syndrome as an adaptation disease in the sense that it is our protective adaptation mechanisms themselves, over-or underreacting, that harm us — "an excess of defensive or overabundance of submissive bodily reactions." In other words, if we do not respond appropriately to the continuous changes around us, we will suffer negatively from stress.

Dr. Selye identified three distinct phases in the stress syndrome. He termed the initial fight-or-flight reaction,

tion, the "alarm" stage. This is followed by the "resistance" stage, in which the body mechanisms adapt themselves to the stressor. In many ways, resistance is the opposite of the first stage; it is accommodation rather than fight/flight. If exposure to a stressor continues, the body's defence system becomes depleted of "adaptation energy" and suffers sudden collapse in the final "exhaustion" stage.

Dr. Selye sees our responses to stressors as largely predetermined by what he calls "internal conditioning" factors, such as heredity and past experiences. For example, if you are accustomed to living in a tropical country and you move to a country that has not only a colder climate but also a different diet and social customs, you would probably experience stress. Physically, your body would have to adjust to different temperatures, humidity and food. Psychologically, you would have to learn new types of behaviour. It takes a lot of energy to adapt, especially if part of you wants to hold on to the old ways. Much unnecessary energy is wasted in internal conflict.

According to Selye, we inherit at birth a certain amount of "adaptation energy," which we gradually expend in responding to the continual challenges that constitute life. If our responses are not appropriate or if the challenges are too demanding, we exhaust our supply of adaptation energy more quickly. We increase the rate of wear and tear on our bodies, becoming more susceptible to illness, injury and premature aging. Conversely, if we adapt efficiently and smoothly, we have more energy available for aliveness, health and well-being. Dr. Selye concludes: "Adaptability is probably the most distinctive characteristic of life . . . There is perhaps a certain parallelism between the degree of aliveness and the extent of adaptability in every animal and in every [human]."

I mention Dr. Selye's theories on stress at the hormonal and biochemical levels because I have long observed the same mechanisms at work at the level of the psyche. Although I do not regard the "internal conditioning factors" or "adaptation energy" as fixed, as Selye seems to, I totally agree with his view of life as a continual response to the challenge of change, for better or for worse.

"Internal conditioning factors" clearly determine most of our life decisions. They are so compulsive that our vaunted freedom of choice is mostly an illusion. They restrict our adaptability not only on the physiological level but also on the mental and emotional levels.

"Conditioning" in this sense includes likes and dislikes, beliefs (religious, political, and cultural), self-image, experiences, customs, habits, knowledge, education, goals and aspirations. Even though we may not do so consciously, we compare almost every new experience with past experiences, measuring them against our belief systems and our accumulated likes and dislikes. We can rarely see with "new" eyes, like a child. We see what we condition ourselves to see or have been conditioned by others to see.

No matter how learned or worldly-wise we may become, our particular bundle of conditioning factors remains haphazard and limited. These factors are certainly insufficient to furnish us with "truth," yet somehow we all have a strong inner conviction that we "know."

These personal conditioning factors, which constitute a large part of what we regard as "I" (our "self"), are not only extremely compulsive but also self-defensive and self-sustaining. They generally recoil and defend themselves from anything new or unknown. In short, they cause in us a deep-seated resistance to real change. They make us less adaptable and less alive. Your alarm mechanisms are constantly being triggered not only by stressors (things, people or situations) that are indeed harmful but also by those that, based on your conditioning factors, merely appear to be so. From here it is just a short step to seeing as harmful anything that does not accord with what you want, or anything that makes you uncomfortable.

On the psychological level, all forms of conflict produce stress. *The Oxford English Dictionary* defines *conflict* as "distress due to opposition of incompatible wishes." J.D. Krishnamurti, a world-renowned spiritual teacher, defined conflict as "the gap between 'what is' and what we want." In other words, you can suffer stress simply from not knowing which choice to make, from not getting what you want or from not wanting to accept something that has happened in your life ("reality"). Since personal desires and choices are so elevated in our society, it is easy to see that we ourselves create much of our stress and conflict through excessive wanting, or greed.

Any form of conflict is an "adaptation disease" in the sense that there is no smooth adaptation or harmony. As long as you are in conflict, there is a degree of alarm and rigidity; there is distress and suffering in some form. Conflict can be internal (within yourself) or external (between yourself and something or someone else). You can experience conflict within particular levels of your being (within the intellect, for example), as well as between levels (between the intellect and the instincts or emotions).

However it manifests itself, conflict is essentially the same and is not easy to resolve. Each of the contentious parts is supported by its own set of internal conditioning factors. Conflict is rather like a group of people (whether two or two million) fighting heatedly over an issue, with each person absolutely convinced that he or she is "right." There is often compromise, alliances, treaties, suppression, winning, losing, avoidance and procrastination. None of this, however, is resolution. This energy (mostly anger) is therefore trapped, like steam building in a pressure-cooker.

Inevitably, when pressures build up or the balance of power shifts, there is an explosion because the central conflict has remained unresolved. In our own lives, we know that a single incident can sour an entire lifetime. Today, countries are still fighting over events that took place hundreds of years ago because there has never been a true resolution of the conflict, despite many treaties and much passage of time.

The effects of stress are more pervasive and destructive than we generally assume. Suppose you are at a social gathering and are introduced to someone for whom you immediately feel a strong dislike. Being a "reasonable" person, you ignore your emotions and make polite conversation for appearances' sake. The incident is soon forgotten.

This seemingly trivial incident is an example of an adaptation malfunction. Because of your conditioning factors (the person reminds you of someone you dislike or perhaps is not behaving "correctly"), you experience an over-reaction and an unnecessary expenditure of nervous and emotional energy. There is no real threat; there is no need for a defensive reaction.

But the malfunction does not end there. Such (often illogical) feelings and judgements accumulate in your subconscious, reinforcing old patterns and beliefs. They may re-emerge later as strong conviction, "truth" or bigotry. The more power you wield over others, whether in the family or at work, the more these distortions are magnified.

We must also take into consideration the cumulative effect of such stress reactions. In a single day you may experience many reactions of this kind, some stronger than others. For example, you miss the bus and are late for work; someone recklessly cuts in front of your car on the way home; you do not get your expected pay increase; the baby-sitter cancels; someone in the line-up at the post office slows things down because he cannot speak English well; or you lose your job.

Pressure, competition, challenge and constant stimulation are now a normal part of modern urban life, along with drugs, pollution, pornography, long working hours, noise and congestion. At one time, most of these would have been considered unhealthy and undesirable. Now they are accepted as unavoidable facets of modern life. This is the resistance stage of the stress syndrome, in which we accommodate our stressors. As we accustom ourselves to each new level of stress, however, the pressure threshold is pushed higher and higher. In our complacency and/or resignation, we accept and participate in what was once considered shocking and unacceptable.

Prolonged exposure to stressors in many areas of our lives has led us to the brink of the final (exhaustion) stage of the stress syndrome — complete and sudden breakdown. There is an ever-increasing incidence of serious physical and mental illness due to nonspecific causes, the trademark of stress. Tempers are short and violence is rampant.

The sense of crisis is also evident at the collective level. Our economies are in the throes of a major restructuring; our cities are decaying; our planet is in critical condition. There is a growing feeling that we may be reaching the limit, as individuals, as a society, as humankind. We may be running out of both time and options.

The bottom line is that there is a bottom line. There is a limit to how much damage an individual, a relationship, a family, a city, a nation, a race, an ocean or a planet can take. Once we become complacent, allowing ourselves to drift or to be pushed to the exhaustion stage, widespread and rapid disintegration is likely. At that stage, the damage is not easy to repair and is sometimes fatal. Our efforts are often too little, too late. It is actually not the last straw that breaks the camel's back but the total accumulation of straws over time.

In 1979, Willy Brandt acknowledged as much. In *North–South: A Program for Survival*, the report of a commission on international development, he warned: "Mankind has never before had such ample technical and financial resources for coping with hunger and poverty. The immense task can be tackled once the necessary collective will is mobilized. What is necessary can be done, and must be done." The problem is not the lack of knowledge or resources but the misuse and abuse of these. Almost all of our major problems are self-inflicted, even many of the ones we think of as "natural disasters." The continuing cycle of drought and starvation in Ethiopia is caused not so much by the lack of rainfall as by a debilitating civil war and the unforgiving realities of Third World economics. The people are not permitted to care for their land, so it turns to dust.

The mobilization of the collective will — that is, a fundamental change in our attitudes to each other — cannot be imposed from the outside, either by force or by persuasion, which includes propaganda and education. In this century, both the Soviet Union and China have made mighty and ruthless efforts to radically remould their citizens. They failed. Even millions of executions could not change the hearts and minds of their people.

For every problem area, there are tomes of intelligent suggestions. The stumbling block to implementation, however, is always the same: ourselves, the very "collective will" Brandt wrote of. If only we were not so selfish, if only we were not so violent, if only we could be more tolerant . . . We fall back on hope, hope that someone, something, some technology or some new consciousness will suddenly arise to save us.

Unfortunately, hope by itself is not enough. We need to do things in a fundamentally different way; we need real change. If we keep on approaching our problems in the same old ways, we will continue to make the same old mistakes.

Mobilizing the Will to Change

How can you break free of your conditioning so that you can respond appropriately to life's movement? It is obvious that you must first understand your conditioning and its source. To do so, you must look within. There can be no other way.

The mind is the source of all internal activity. It triggers mechanisms at all levels — physical, emotional, mental and spiritual. Before you can feel threatened, wronged or pressured, you must first have an idea of who you are, what your rights are and what another person's actions or words mean to you. In order to perform any conscious activity, you must have the desire to do it and an idea of how it should be done.

Much of our "external" environment and stressors are created by the "internal" mind. Buildings, roads, cars, pollution, television, drugs and weapons are not just given materials of life. They were conceived and produced by our collective mind operating under the direction of our collective internal conditioning factors. "Internal" and "external" are therefore mutually conditioning and interdependent.

Not only is the external ultimately determined by the internal, but the collective is determined by the individual. The collective will is nothing more than the accumulation of our individual desires and actions. The seemingly impersonal forces of technology, economics and government that fashion our lives are actually the work of mortal, fallible, confused people like you and me — scientists, politicians, image manipulators and bureaucrats.

Although these "remote" forces shape us, we in turn shape them. They are influenced by what we think, how we vote, what we buy and even how we dispose of our garbage. All the symptoms that we see in our society — polarization, isolation, alienation, depersonalization, the increase of violence — are also to be found in our individual lives. This is not a coincidence.

Individual transformation as the source of collective transformation is as remarkably obvious as it is exciting. It means that there is something, after all, that we can do for our planet. Moreover, that something is no different from what we urgently need to do for our individual well-being. Rather than being paralysed by the thought of the Thousand-Mile Journey ahead of us, we can take the first step, which is always here and now.

Hans Selye's work at the biochemical level led him also to the mind as the logical source of efficient adaptation: "The ancient Greek philosophers clearly recognized that, with regard to human conduct, the most important, but perhaps also the most difficult, thing was 'to know thyself' . . . Yet it is well worth the effort and humiliation, because most of our tensions and frustrations stem from compulsive needs to act the role of someone we are not."

"To know thyself" is indeed difficult. It is difficult because our "self" does not want to be known. Our sense of "self" or "I" consists largely of the very internal conditioning factors from which we are trying to free ourselves. When we attempt to change them, one part of the "I" is, in effect, coercing another. This is akin to trying to lift yourself up by your own bootstraps. Thus, even "sensible" changes, like eliminating pollution, drug abuse, torture, wars and starvation, are difficult to accomplish.

The major prerequisite for real change is to see clearly the urgent necessity for it and to take the first step. You need not stumble to the edge of the precipice in order to acquire a sense of urgency. You have only to open your eyes unconditionally to what is going on in your life now. If you do, you will spot the precipice in plenty of time to take evasive action.

For myself, the external change from chartered accountant to teacher of Insight Meditation and the martial arts was only the spark of a transformational flame. Change reached into all areas and levels of my life — physical, emotional, intellectual and spiritual; it burned away much dead wood and transformed all my relationships so that the new — simple, joyous and creative — could emerge.

Much of the change was undramatic but invaluable. My first experience of what I would call real change occurred when I was training to be a chartered accountant. The work was tedious, and anyhow I could not see myself as an accountant for life. Yet it was the "safe and reasonable" thing to do and I should have considered myself fortunate. Like so many others, I was torn and in conflict, doing something I did not really want to do. I looked forward to coffee and lunch breaks, to the end of the day, to weekends and to holidays, but they were never enough to compensate me for the daily grind. I began to find fault in everything and everyone around me; I was irritable and restless.

Increasingly discontented, I decided to apply my rudimentary meditation practice to "real life." Seeking "clear comprehension of purpose," I finally "saw" (with more than just the intellect) that while accounting was indeed limited and not something to which I wanted to devote my life, there was nothing else at that time that I really wanted to do or was indeed qualified to do. It was clear that I had been fighting myself for no good reason and causing my own suffering.

Having fully accepted the suitability of what I was doing, my struggles immediately subsided. The job was exactly the same, but I was transformed. I derived satisfaction from doing the job for its own sake; I no longer watched the clock, and consequently time flew by; I was able to leave my job preoccupations at the office and fully enjoy my leisure time. For the first time in my life, I could let go of unnecessary and inappropriate concerns and ideas and begin living moment by moment.

Freeing ourselves from our conditioning — achieving real change — is what this book is all about. It is not easy, but it can be done, and indeed must be done, if we are to bring about the radical change in attitude that both Einstein and Brandt called for. If we can successfully meet the challenges of life, moment to moment, then we will have learnt the invaluable lesson of how, in the words of the *Tao Te Ching*, to "manage the great while they are small." A crisis becomes a crisis only because matters get out of hand. If we attend to minor problems, they do not become major ones. Taking one step at a time, never attempting the great, we can walk the Thousand-Mile Journey; we can achieve the great.

II

WHY REAL CHANGE IS RARE

"How can a mind that is fearful, envious, acquisitive, discover that which is beyond itself? It will find only its own projections — the images, beliefs and conclusions in which it is caught."
— *J.D. KRISHNAMURTI*

"The object of every right desire is within our reach, though unseen, concealed by a veil of illusion. As one not knowing that a golden treasure lies buried beneath his feet, may walk over it again and again, yet never find it, so all beings live every moment in the city of Brahman, yet never find him."
— *THE UPANISHADS*

Whenever I speak of the need for real change, people often get defensive and irate. I am often asked the same questions: "What's wrong with me the way I am?" "Aren't we changing all the time anyway?" "Haven't we progressed?" "Aren't we learning from experience and making discoveries?" "Isn't this or that scientific/psychological/spiritual technique the answer?" To me, the intensity of this reaction is itself a demonstration of people's resistance to change — in this case, merely the notion of a different approach to life. *Why* are we so resistant?

Our environment is changing rapidly. Runaway science and technology have given us enormous power, but as Einstein observed, there has been no corresponding increase in our wisdom to use that power. In other words, our intellectual development is out of balance with our stunted emotional and spiritual growth. It is frightening that world leaders can state their philosophy proudly as "Speak softly and carry a big stick" and not raise many eyebrows, especially when the "big stick" in question is the power to destroy whole countries or perhaps even civilization as we know it.

Despite our ingenious rationalizations and justifications, the motivation for our actions ultimately comes down to "me first" — me, my family, my job, my neighbourhood, my social class, my race, my country, my religion, my ideology. We cannot justify our actions logically on the grounds of our "natural" instinct for self-preservation since we rarely face life-threatening situations. We may be better or worse off than others, but that is hardly a matter of self-preservation. Some of the most aggressive and acquisitive people in our society are already the most rich and powerful.

We usually try to soften the effect of "me first" with the idea of charity. The thinking goes, "When I have accumulated enough money or power to feel secure, then I will share my surplus." That was more or less the rationale behind the Reagan and Thatcher doctrines of the 1980s. The fact is, we never have enough to feel secure. Since the 1960s, the gap between rich and poor (and the envy and anger it generates) has been increasing. It always amazes me that rich and poor alike try to convince themselves that a healthy, cohesive society could be built on the divisiveness of greed.

Attaining our "me first" goals usually means using others. My dictionary defines *use* as "cause to act or serve for a purpose, handle as instrument, consume as material, exercise, put into operation, avail oneself of." Others become secondary — instruments to our purpose. The element of exploitation is obvious in all our relationships, whether with other humans, with other countries or cultures, with other animal species or with our environment. We invariably want to be in control. We forget that for every "success," controller, exploiter, superior, there is the failure, the controlled, the exploited, the inferior. The second group far outnumbers the first.

Apart from the destructive credo of "me first," our power to manipulate our environment has not brought the benefits that we expected. In the West, the material standard of living has sky-rocketed in this century, but it is debatable whether we are any happier or any more secure than our forebears or those who live in "underdeveloped" countries. When I travelled through rural India, peasants considered themselves fortunate to have a week's supply of food. Indeed, they were eager to share it with me.

The real costs of the "comfort and convenience" that we have been pursuing are only now becoming apparent. Our lives grow ever more hectic and, in many ways, less healthy. On some days, for example, we are cautioned to stay indoors because the very air we breathe or the sun that otherwise gives us life is considered harmful; many lakes and rivers are no more than glorified sewers; it is almost impossible to buy food free of toxins or chemicals; something as basic as getting to and from work results in extreme stress.

The more power we wield, the greater is the risk of catastrophic error, either of commission or omission. The more we bring under our control, the more there is to slip out of control. As Willy Brandt wrote, we already have ample power. What we need to develop is the ability to use it constructively.

Progress, Reform and Fragmentation

Time, experience and "progress" are not the automatic answers to our problems that we assume. If we really did learn as much as we think we do, then older people would necessarily be wiser, which is plainly not the case. Our historical lessons have been repeated so often, we should have graduated to Utopia long ago. We always seem to be progressing, accumulating possessions and knowledge, yet never quite reaching our destination, never having quite enough. There is always more to be done and more to struggle for, no matter how much success we may have enjoyed in the past. It never seems to occur to us that this is not bad luck, but an inherent flaw in how we conceive of life.

Although the ideals of progress and hope are almost sacrosanct in our society, they can be an impediment. If you think you are making progress and that things will be all right no matter what, then you will lack a sense of urgency. You will take no immediate and decisive action. You will have no spirit of enquiry. You will tolerate what ought to be intolerable. In the terminology of stress, you will be in the "resistance" stage, wherein you accommodate yourself to something that is harming you. Most people abhor starvation, wars and torture, yet these exist not only in our world but are widespread. Some studies estimate that more than half of the world's governments use torture as an instrument of policy. The destruction of our planet (and by necessity ourselves) through environmental abuse is in danger of becoming just another "issue" or "cause." We accept air and sunlight hazard warnings unquestioningly, as facts of life, as if they had nothing to do with human decisions and actions — *our* decisions and actions. We should be outraged and alarmed. We are not . . . yet.

This same complacency exists on the individual level. It is common for people to remain in abusive work or family situations because they hope that better times are just around the corner, that the abuser will change, or because they have simply become accustomed to it. They are afraid to risk the unfamiliar even if the familiar means senseless pain and suffering.

Real change is rare because we usually seek not change but reform. My dictionary defines *change* as "making or becoming different." *Reform* is to "form again" or "make or become better by removal or abandonment of imperfections, faults or errors." Becoming new is a rarely expressed goal in our society. We are usually engrossed in removing imperfections, trying to patch up, cover over, improve or simply snatch some breathing space for ourselves.

The removal of imperfections can be a valid strategy, but we usually attempt to remove not the imperfection itself but only manifestations of it, one by one. This ongoing process can never meet with success. By attempting only piecemeal changes in our lives, we are treating the symptoms, not the disease. This means not only that the untreated disease will worsen but that we are wasting vital resources and often causing unnecessary and damaging complications.

You may, for example, feel a constant need to be admired or complimented, to receive "positive feedback." This may cause you to exhaust yourself trying to please or impress others at work or in one relationship after another; you may attempt to improve your appearance through diet, exercise, clothes or cosmetic surgery; if things are not going well, you may seek solace in food, drink, sex or drugs.

True independence and self-esteem, however, can arise only from within yourself. No matter what you do, you will never be able to control what other people think and feel about you. The innumerable ways of trying to escape or cover over problems will be in vain as long as the root cause remains.

Another reason we adopt a piecemeal approach to change is because that is how we perceive life. We divide life into countless conceptual boxes, for example, work, family, health and leisure. The more information we generate, however, the more complicated each box becomes and the more boxes we have to maintain. We become indecisive, confused, overburdened. Right now, we are inundated with information about the various mechanisms of the body and mind. To cite just one example, every day we hear about new recommended diets and exercises of a physical, mental and spiritual nature. Although much of this information is valid, it remains limited and fragmentary. We still do not know how to choose what is true or relevant for us or how to make all the conceptual parts fit together as a whole. In the end, we remain frustrated and confused, frantically trying one diet or exercise after another.

In reality, body, mind and energy do not exist separately. They are part of an integrated, inseparable and continually changing whole. It is only our intellect that perceives them as separate and distinct. Ironically, we continue trying to find wholeness through the very process that causes us to feel unwhole and fragmented — intellectualizing. The human embodiment of the intellect, the specialist, will tell you about his or her particular specialty but not about how to integrate it into a whole. This is the greater problem.

Naturally, this same fragmentation is evident in our collective lives. There are always new and pressing issues for society and government to confront.

We are generally strong on analyses and recommendations, but weak on achieving real change. Whether the issue is discrimination, violence, the environment, the military, the economy, drugs, AIDS, immigration, welfare or global relationships, the recommendations and actions generally fall into three categories: form or join a pressure group or political party to push your particular issue; enact new legislation or regulations; or obtain money for funding, research and education. We assume that these are the only ways to get things done, whether we see ourselves as part of the establishment or outside of it. (Political "revolution" usually entails the same process, except it is more violent, spans a broader spectrum of issues and takes place over a longer time.)

But an examination of these approaches, as applied to various issues and over various periods, reveals four failings.

First, they are ineffective and inefficient. There is an enormous expenditure of time, energy and money, and one can always cite examples of "progress," but the major problem remains, in one form or another. Our eagerness for immediate, "decisive" action covers our ignorance about what truly needs to be done; the short term takes precedence over the long term.

Second, one "just cause" is invariably in competition with another for limited resources and public sympathy. Sometimes, just causes are in direct opposition to each other.

Third, organizations responsible for "solving" a problem often have a conscious or subconscious interest in prolonging the problem. After all, no more problem means no more job and no more recognition.

And fourth, special interests usually generate further special interests, and thus more fragmentation.

Analysis creates more parts; it does not put them together. Our lives, both on the individual and collective levels, urgently need a healing, integrative force to counteract the slide towards division and fragmentation. It is imperative that we find a source of integration before we fall apart completely.

The Blind-Spot

"Unseen, but the seer; unheard, but the hearer; unthinkable, but the thinker; unknown, but the knower — there is no other seer but he, no other hearer but he, no other thinker but he, no other knower but he. He,

the Self,* is the Inner Ruler, the Immortal. Anything that is not the Self perishes."

— THE UPANISHADS

There is a blind-spot in our consciousness. It keeps us from truly learning from our experience, from bridging the gap between what we know needs to be done and doing it and from finding wholeness, harmony and contentment. It keeps us locked in a vicious circle of suffering.

That blind-spot is ourselves. All thoughts and activities flow from the centre that we identify as our "I," our "self." We are the willing slaves of a host of inner voices and urges, yet we know very little about them — about where they come from, about which voice to believe. Our "I" seems solid and real enough, yet if we look for it, it is nowhere to be found. It is neither a limb nor an organ; it is not even the brain.

We tend to ignore this blind-spot because it is the Unknown — inexplicable, threatening, uncontrollable, potentially chaotic. It is common to hear people say, "It is better not to delve too deeply into things, not to think too much, not to stir things up." Such statements reflect both a recognition (not necessarily conscious) and a fear of what truly underlies our conventional "realities."

No matter what or how hard you try, your efforts will not contribute to your deeper well-being if you do not know who you really are and what you really need. (Short-term success in getting what you *want* is not the same as getting what you *need.*) In turn, you cannot find this out unless you pose the question with skill and

---

* "Self" in this sense is Brahman, God, the source of all manifestation. When we get lost in our identity of the little or separate egoic self (the "I"), we lose the sense of the greater Self and Oneness — our true source and identity.

perseverance. Not knowing yourself, you are forced to repeat your patterns again and again, despite whatever pain they may cause you.

Self-knowledge is not automatically accumulated like your knowledge of the world around you. The blind-spot moves with the looker so that although the field of vision changes, self-knowledge remains hidden. Think of the universe as a room. If you want to know all you can about that room, you would first look around you. There will be some parts of the room you cannot immediately see, so you keep changing your perspective until you feel you have covered every nook and cranny. You will then feel your knowledge is complete; you "know" that room; there is no need for further enquiry. The one thing that will have escaped you, however, is the most important part: you, the looker.

Even if attention is turned inside, one part of yourself is usually looking at another, and the looker still remains hidden and separate. Thus, it is possible for meditators to encounter unusual, fascinating inner experiences and even extraordinary powers, yet learn very little about the meditator. Outside of their periods of meditation and inner work, their lives and problems often remain the same or may even worsen as they compare their lofty spiritual experiences with the seeming banality and pointlessness of their everyday lives.

Some people look inside and conclude, quite rightly, that the answer to their problems is love and self-lessness. If this conclusion is just intellectual, however, it will not in itself resolve their problems. It would still not bridge that frustrating gap between where they are (me first) and where they want to be (selfless and loving), between what needs doing and what is done. I once saw a car bumper sticker that proclaimed, "Jesus loves you . . . and I am trying to."

What makes this blind-spot even more difficult to grasp is that it is not just one entity. Our ego or "I" is like a shell or structure inhabited by a great number of patterns or sub-personalities, each jostling for a turn to express itself. There may be the parent, the child, the man or woman, the careerist, the sage, the shadow, the helper, the savage, the worrier, the bully, the coward, the prankster, and many more. These sub-personalities may be likened to many people inhabiting the same body. When we say "I feel there is a battle going on inside myself," we are often nearer the truth than we realize.

These sub-personalities and patterns constitute in large measure the internal conditioning factors that Hans Selye identified as determining our responses to life.

Because we are unaware of this vast blind-spot and because we are rarely able to change our deep patterns, we think of ourselves as fixed and unchanging. Not only do we regard our internal conditioning factors as given, but we routinely exult in the fact of our conditioning. Patriotism, racism, religion, history and even individuality ("I'm proud to be me and I don't want to change!") are often simply excuses to justify conditioned behaviour. Bigotry is an extreme form of this mechanism.

Having accepted ourselves as solid and unchanging, we direct most of our activity outward. We try to change other people or our environment to suit ourselves; we look to others — including God, gurus, philosophers and experts — for wisdom, advice, expertise, something to believe in; we look to others to fill us up, keep us company, reassure us and make us feel secure.

The goal of all our attempts at change, and indeed of everything we do, is security. We feel solid, but never solid enough. There is always an underlying fear, a fear of not having or being enough, of losing what we have, of the unknown, of the unexpected and of death. Our deepest fear is of the Unknown in all its forms, including Death, the Void, Chaos and Madness. We fear it because we cannot know it and therefore cannot predict it or control it. We seek reassurance in money, fame, power, belief and "spirituality"; we seek to possess people, things or ideas; we expand with the sense of achievement, of being needed, of being desirable, of being part of a band of true believers.

We pursue all these things in order to feel more substantial, more real. We reassure ourselves that if all these things are solid (and they seem to be because other people accept them as such), and we can possess them or have some relationship with them, then we too must be solid. These attachments help us build and fortify the walls and structures that the ego or "I" uses to keep its fears at bay.

The biggest flaw in our ego defence plan is that the Unknown is not outside our ramparts but is lurking within. Wherever we go, it goes. It does not matter how much power or knowledge we have accumulated or what we have achieved, it is never enough. At our core, we are insubstantial, insufficient and incomplete. (If we were complete, most of our present activities would be redundant.). We can never make our "self" solid because it is not solid and never has been.

The Buddha expressed the human dilemma in terms of attachment. The second of his Four Noble Truths states that we suffer because we try to attach or hold on to life (or to push it away, which is the negative aspect of holding) when there is nothing that can be held. He saw life as impermanent and in a constant state of flux — bundles of creative activities giving rise to each other. Consequently, whenever we try to hold on to life, it slips through our fingers like sand. We feel this loss as suffering, because we can never be truly satisfied and content.

Twenty-five hundred years later, subatomic physics is giving scientific validation to the Buddha's insight into the nature of the universe. We are now being told that the universe is not a collection of solid objects travelling through absolute time and space. It is rather a vast, interconnected and ever-changing web of energy relationships, impermanent and insubstantial. If nothing in the universe is solid, it follows that neither are we. Yet we continue to feel so.

Although these scientific theories are taught in schools and are widely applied within society, we do not apply them to ourselves. We still see ourselves as separate islands travelling through time and space. Separateness is still the basis of our legal, economic and social systems. This omission should come as no surprise. It is the manifestation of our collective blind-spot, our disregard of the obvious.

The Universal Dilemma

The blind-spot in our consciousness is not my discovery or invention. Most of the great religions and philosophies have alluded to it in one way or another. It is a universal dilemma that arose with the evolution of our mental ego-consciousness, the sense of separate self.

In the Christian tradition, it is implied in the story of Adam and Eve eating the fruit from the Tree of Knowledge. Before eating the fruit, Adam and Eve were as innocent as animals or babies. There was no sense of separation in space or in time. Everything was totally and timelessly present. As soon as they ate the fruit and developed the power to discriminate good from evil, they became separate — from God, from each other, from animals, and from their environment. They also experienced temporal separation for the first time and began the inevitable journey towards death. They were banished from their paradise of innocence: "Then the Lord said, 'Now that the man has become as we are, knowing good from bad, what if he eats from the Tree of Life and lives forever?' So the Lord God banished him forever from the Garden of Eden, and sent him out to farm the ground from which he had been taken. Thus God expelled him, and placed mighty angels . . . to guard the entrance to the Tree of Life."

The *Tao Te Ching* (written in China in the third to fourth century B.C.) and *The Upanishads* (written in India in the seventh century B.C.) describe the same dilemma but from a different perspective.

> *"From eternal nonexistence, we serenely observe the mysterious beginning of the Universe;*
> *From eternal existence we clearly see the apparent distinctions.*
> *These two are the same in source and become different when manifested . . .*
> *When all the world understand beauty to be beautiful, then ugliness exists.*
> *When all understand goodness to be good, then evil exists.*
> *Thus existence suggests nonexistence;*
> *Easy gives rise to difficult."*
> — THE TAO TE CHING

> *"As long as there is duality, one sees the other, one hears the other, one smells the other, one speaks to the other, one thinks of the other, one knows the other; but when for the illumined soul the all is dissolved in Self, who is there to be seen by whom?"*
> — THE UPANISHADS

The intellect is a double-edged sword. On one side, it confers on us the exhilaration of being individual, unique and able to wield power. It enables us to analyse and break things down into their component parts so that we can study and manipulate them. It is the basis of modern society's enormous power to manipulate the environment.

On the other side, it makes us separate, divided, vulnerable, insecure and mortal. It cuts off the individual from the rest of the universe (all that is not the "I"), which is the very ground of our being. It is the cause of conflict, strife and wars.

Since this division and fragmentation also takes place within, it separates one part of the self from another. Thus, one part of us may be "good" and another "evil"; one may be "deep" and another "superficial"; one may be "true" and another "false." Often these disparate parts are in conflict. Since we have little insight into the real nature of our conflicts, we can rarely resolve them; we remain caught. We can rarely experience real change within ourselves.

In truth, a wholeness always underlies all the separate parts that we discern. We have, however, become blind to it and see only the differences. We need to regain our sight; we need "in-sight" into the Oneness of our deeper self.

The yin-yang symbol is a depiction of the universe that reconciles the apparent contradictions between the opposites and between duality and oneness. This symbol represents all pairs of opposites: female/male, heaven/earth, good/bad, black/white, inner/outer, the head/heart, and so on. These polarities, however, are interdependent. They do not stand in eternal opposition to each other as, for example, do the Christian concepts of God and the Devil. Yin contains an element of yang, and vice versa. Extreme yin becomes yang and extreme yang returns to yin. Yin and yang are always seeking to balance each other.

The circle represents the Tao, the Unconditioned, the ultimate Source out of which yin and yang arose. This Tao both precedes yin and yang and includes their continuous interplay. It was and continues to be their source.

As long as our "I" sees itself only as a separate, independent entity (in other words, only as yin or yang), it will be cut off from its true nature and source — the Tao, the original Oneness. It will be in a perpetual state of disharmony or imbalance, fighting a hopeless and necessarily losing battle to safeguard itself from the flow of the universe, which it regards as separate from itself, the "non-I."

There is no psychological, financial or other kind of strategy that ever has or ever will guarantee the ego its security. There is nothing to which the "I" can really cling, whether people, material possessions, ideas or even religious beliefs. This needless struggle exhausts many of us long before death claims us. We go through the mere motions of life.

Real change means responding to the ceaseless interplay of yin and yang, to the movements of the Tao or universe. Our "I," on the other hand, is usually trying its utmost to arrest real change. It is comprehensively conditioned, with fixed ideas of who it is and how life should be. It is always trying to feel solid in order to avoid admitting the possibility that it is in fact as insubstantial and changeable as everything else in the universe.

Much stress and anxiety, even wars, are caused by our inability and unwillingness to accept that life is changing all the time. This is what the Buddha meant when he pointed out that all suffering is caused by attachment. If we are not attached, then even death loses its sting. It becomes merely another experience, another moment, another challenge, another movement of the Tao. I must point out that "nonattachment" in this sense is not the lack of caring or doing, merely the absence of grasping. We can live zestfully without needing or expecting to hold on to the good times.

The universal dilemma we all face is how to change the source of our actions from duality ("I" and "me first" consciousness) when the "I" is now in control (it is reading this book right now). The "I" is a tyrant that will

35

not willingly give up its power. It is afraid of losing control, of admitting past mistakes, of being engulfed and swept away, of being put to death. This fear, which results from the ignorance of its own true nature (the Self, the Tao, the Source, the Unconditioned), is extremely deep and keeps us trapped in our suffering; it keeps us from changing at deeper levels.

The "I" cannot change itself. It can only let go of its need to control and allow itself to be changed and made whole. This may sound depressing and threatening, but it follows that a fragment (your "I") cannot make itself the whole merely by altering its boundaries or creating further fragments.

As soon as you say "My present state is so-and-so, but I need to be over there," you create more distance, you create another fragment. Loving is not the same as trying to love; being simple is not the same as trying to be simple; being whole is not the same as trying to be whole. Everyone makes "progress," but usually there is still something lacking, something else to rectify or improve. Rather than accepting this as human nature, we need to explore how this feeling of incompleteness arises in us and how it shapes our lives.

It is human destiny that we will one day see our Oneness just as clearly as we now see our separateness. The words *universal brotherhood* and *the global family* will be more than noble sentiments that are discarded when we get down to the bottom line — me versus you, my family versus yours, my nation or god versus yours.

That next step in the evolution of human consciousness will come sooner or later. The question with which we must concern ourselves is how bad do things have to get before we are forced to do what we must do anyway. Thousands of years are nothing in human history. Yet right now we can ill afford to make any more major mistakes in managing our collective lives and that of our planet. Right now many of us can ill afford to make one more major mistake concerning our individual health and well-being. A lifespan of sixty or eighty years is relatively fleeting. It amounts to a handful of major relationships, jobs and belief systems. We do not have that many opportunities to get it "right."

In spite of the hope that a new age of consciousness is dawning, we cannot expect the average human consciousness to make a quantum leap within the next fifty years and remedy all our problems for us. Right now, we badly need real change. This can come about only by individual change. Change cannot be legislated, educated or implemented by force. The odds may be against our making an individual leap in consciousness, but if we can clearly see the necessity for real change within ourselves, it will be the start of a process. We at least give ourselves the chance to become a statistical improbability and, as the nuclear-power industry will attest, statistical improbabilities can and do occur all the time.

What Is Real Change?

Like Hans Selye, I associate aliveness with adaptability. I have tried to show that on many levels we are not nearly as adaptable as we think. This severely affects our aliveness and our well-being, individually and as a society.

If you were literally fighting for your life, against a tiger for example, adaptability would clearly be the key to your survival. You would not know what to expect; you would not be able to predict the tiger's actions. If you allowed yourself to be paralysed by fear, not only would you be incapable of physical response but your fear itself might trigger an attack. If you adopted a rigid strategy such as attacking first, running or shouting, you might likewise worsen your predicament.

Your best chance would lie in being totally alert, ready for action, but quiet, like the tiger itself. Too many ideas can confuse you. This may be a chance encounter and the tiger may be as startled as you are; perhaps the tiger is testing your nerve or will to fight; maybe it is intent on attack. Your survival would depend on your (adapt)ability in being able to read the situation and to respond appropriately. Overreaction could be as disastrous as underreaction. You could die from an "adaptation malfunction."

It is exactly the same in the martial arts. A weaponless, no-rules fight demands total response. Not only are strength and speed required but so too are courage, sensitivity and flexibility of both body and mind. The key to such a response is not the body, as we might imagine, but the mind.

Total response arises out of complete emptiness. If the mind and body are distracted or impeded in any way, then the response cannot be total and appropriate. Often too much effort results in less speed and power; likewise too much thinking can result in confusion, inappropriate response, or even paralysis. This excerpt from the Tai Chi Chuan classics describes the state of internal equilibrium necessary for effective martial response: "We are centred, stable and still as a mountain. Our Chi [internal energy] sinks to the Tan Tien [just below the navel] and our torso is as if suspended from above. Our spirit is concentrated within and our outward manner perfectly composed. Receiving and issuing energy are both the work of an instant."

We can see many of these same mechanisms at work in the more familiar context of sport. In tennis and baseball, games that are almost as much mental as physical, the exceptional players are those who can let go of the bad play or game, who can continually match an opponent's change in tactics, and who can concentrate on the essential simplicity of what they are doing — see ball, hit ball. Frank Boehm, a noted sports psychologist, explained, "A sports psychologist has the best results by helping a person focus on the actual task that's to be performed. Kicking a field goal really means kicking the ball between the upright poles; scoring is secondary."

Such players are not invincible, but they are much less prone to slumps and self-doubt, to abuse of their bodies and minds and to self-defeat. Their consistency and flexibility, products of a superior mental attitude rather than of physical skills, give them longevity and prominence in their chosen sport.

The tiger, the martial arts and the ball game are life itself. They are dramatic and simplified illustrations of the challenges we face in everyday life. The particular tiger in your life could be your health, boss, lover, job, or a deceptively "harmless" habit or foible. You must be totally present and totally aware of all the changing circumstances, internally and externally, in order to respond to this challenge.

Unfortunately, we are rarely in touch with the present because our response is almost always dictated by old patterns, beliefs and hopes. Our past conditioning exerts a continuous push-pull force on us. We compare all experiences with past experiences, beliefs and patterns. These "push" us by determining our responses to the present. The effects of these responses, in turn, condition the future by determining what options are open to us. We enhance this "pull" effect by our expectations and aspirations, all of which are projected from the past. We are, therefore, continually responding to the present from the past, a process that is inappropriate, limiting and sometimes disastrous.

From the present standpoint of the "I," the concept of just being in the moment is not only difficult to understand but also threatening. This is because the main function of the "I" is to continue its own existence. It does this by an almost uninterrupted process of "becoming" — physically or mentally going somewhere or doing something. It is difficult for the "I" just "to be" because it ceases to exist in the state of just being. There is no "I" during dreamless sleep; there is no "I" without thinking. If you suffered from amnesia, your familiar "I" would be lost.

People who attend my courses and talks find them interesting and thought-provoking, but they often voice reservations such as, "If we didn't have goals, we would become vegetables. We would be pushed around and life would become chaotic"; "We must have beliefs or else we would be nothing or would degenerate into animals"; "Belief in God is the foundation of life"; "These theories sound fine, but real life is different"; "Wouldn't we all become robots, thinking and acting the same?"

These objections reflect some of the fundamental fears and mechanisms of the "I." We like to have beliefs and goals because they keep us engrossed in the process of "becoming." The business of projecting ourselves into the future keeps us busy and stimulated; it also helps cover over (but not resolve) any discomfort and emptiness in the present.

Belief is one of our main ego-defence mechanisms. The belief that you must have belief and goals is just that — a belief. Your belief is not the truth, no matter how many other people share it. You can undoubtedly use your beliefs to fortify your sense of self, but in so doing, you wall yourself in and create a siege mentality.

The stronger your belief, the more you are compelled to defend it, because the more you are identified with it. It is you. When your beliefs are threatened, you are threatened. That is why people kill and are killed for their beliefs, convinced that God, Truth and even Love must be on their side. Belief in this sense is psychological self-defence, which must be distinguished from physical self-defence, as when your person or country is physically attacked.

Beliefs and goals are fundamental elements in the push-pull of conditioning. The past gives us security and a feeling of control because it is the known. We try to maintain this security by projecting it into the future in the guise of goals, aspirations and planning. All the past, all the experience and the knowledge are us, the "I," and as such we are identified with them. We are driven to perpetuate this accumulation of patterns, so if they are threatened, we will defend them, and we will defend even those that are destroying us. We are haunted by the spectre of emptiness, of not being, of the unknown — which in many cases obscures the real damage we are inflicting on ourselves.

These conditioning mechanisms, which most of us would regard as human nature, give the lie to our self-concepts of open-mindedness and rationality. Most of us are not really interested in exploring the new, but are searching for different ways of expressing or propping up what we already believe and do. If we were really open-minded, we would not be threatened or upset by ideas that disagreed with our fundamental premises. We generally seek reassurance rather than truth. The more people (or the "right" type of people) that believe as we do, the more secure we feel. However, truth has nothing to do with quantity or with security.

To me, real change means the ability to respond to each moment as a new moment. To do this we must be awake and alert, free to perceive what response is required and free to carry out that response. Real change is responding to life as it is rather than struggling to cram it into our own narrow range of expectations and patterns of response. It is openness, softness and fluidity rather than contraction and rigidity. The *Tao Te Ching*, pre-dating Hans Selye by more than two and a half thousand years, notes, "All plants and animals when living are tender and fragile; when dead they become withered and dry."

If you centre yourself in the present, life will become simpler, more harmonious and more integrated. Deep insight into the present moment not only frees you from past patterns but allows you to respond fully to the present. Effective response in the present is in turn the best course of action that you can take to avoid future complications and difficulties. Therefore, instead of worrying about the past or the future, you must, like the ball player, give full attention to the present moment. Tom Seaver, now a Hall of Fame baseball pitcher, once observed, "As I refine my pitching, I am refining the pleasure I get from it. A victory used to give me pleasure, then a well-pitched inning, and now I get satisfaction from just one or two pitches a game. I get in a situation where I have to apply all I know, mentally and physically, in just one pitch."

Through insight into the present moment, you can resolve your deep conflicts and experience harmony and integration in many unexpected ways. Since all aspects of your being are interdependent, resolution of conflict will affect not only all the manifestations of that particular conflict but all levels of your being — physical, emotional, mental, and so on.

I once witnessed a rather dramatic example of this unravelling at Dhiravamsa's meditation retreat centre in England. One of my fellow meditators noticed that he was leaning to one side during his sitting meditations with the group. Being an experienced meditator, he attributed this to tiredness and resolved to sit upright, as he thought an experienced meditator should. His determination brought about an improvement in his posture, although he still experienced a slight tugging sensation at his side. Following one of Dhiravamsa's talks on the need to be compassionate with oneself, he decided to let go of his image of being an experienced meditator and to let himself be taken wherever the tugging wanted to take him.

The most terrifying scream I have ever heard shattered the quiet of that English summer evening. The man fell to his side, convulsing, shrieking, coughing, sputtering as he went into a foetal position. This went on for nearly an hour before the screaming gradually turned to laughter from relief and joy. It turned out he had relived a near-drowning experience (confirmed by a call to his grandmother) dating from before the age of two, even to the extent of regurgitating what he said tasted like seawater.

Many things fell into place for the man that evening. Many of his life-long problems with his body, with his relationships, with his jobs and with life in general could be traced back to this single experience. It explained why, when life became difficult, he felt overwhelmed, pushed under and suffocated. Suddenly, both his body and his psyche felt lighter and freer.

Merely by allowing and paying close attention to something that seemed ordinary and insignificant (the tugging), he suddenly understood and experienced liberation from many seemingly unconnected problems in his life. Moreover, he had now experienced the mechanisms and the power of real change. It was a new beginning for him, not only in the sense of letting go of a great burden from the past but of being able to face the ongoing challenges of life in a completely different manner.

Although real change is rare and is our biggest challenge, it is also ordinary and everyday. It is getting up each day and making your way through the rush-hour; it is work; it is your family; it is birth, death, joy and grief. All the little things, as well as the more dramatic, you can see differently, you can do differently. You can make space within yourself for understanding and compassion to grow, and in time you can enjoy the fruits of your labours. All this must be done not with the expectation of the fruit, but because there is no other choice. Your eyes are finally wide open and you simply do what you see you must.

The Thousand-Mile Journey starts with the spot beneath our feet and is accomplished one step at a time. This is so obvious that it is often overlooked. We can in fact take only one step at a time, no matter how exhilarating or painful the journey seems at that time. The present moment is the only moment for action — not the past or the future. If we do not wake up and pay attention to each step, we may become overwhelmed and discouraged by the distance ahead or by our present difficulties. We may stumble and injure ourselves. If, on the other hand, we do pay attention to each step, we can avoid pitfalls and will indeed journey far.

III

TRANSFORMATION: OPENING TO THE NEW

"Be free from the future; be free of the past; be free in the present; cross to the yonder shore. With a mind wholly free, you will not fall into birth and death."
— THE DHAMMAPADA, COLLECTED SAYINGS OF THE BUDDHA.

"The most beautiful and profound emotion we can experience is the sensation of the mystical. It is the true sower of all art and science. He to whom this emotion is a stranger, who can no longer wonder and stand rapt in awe, is as good as dead."
— *ALBERT EINSTEIN*

You cannot open to the new — you cannot experience real change and creativity — if you are bound by the old. The new is the present moment. The old is the past — memories, beliefs, patterns, likes and dislikes. Surprisingly, the future is also the old, since it is merely a mental projection based on your past experiences.

The present moment is also the only real opportunity you have for action. You can never act in the past or in the future. Both are mental creations; without thinking, neither past nor future exists for us.

All this is indisputable, yet we have become such complex beings that the obvious escapes us. Most of us find it difficult even to imagine the possibility of life without constantly picking over the past and planning or worrying about the future. We are arrogant enough to believe that if we do not control the world, chaos will ensue. Ironically, much of the present chaos in the world has been created by our very efforts to prevent it. Jesus admonished us: "Do not worry about things — food, drink and clothes. For you already have life and a body — and they are far more important than what to eat and wear. Look at the birds! They do not worry about what to eat — they do not need to sow or reap or store up food — for your heavenly Father feeds them. And you are far more valuable to him than they are."

Unfortunately, trying not to worry and trying to be simple do not work. We are already worried and we are already complex. A complex person trying to be simple becomes even more complex. The more ideas we have, the more we are removed from the immediacy of the present.

Each moment of our lives is so powerfully conditioned by the past that the present is almost incidental. As soon as we become conscious of something, we automatically compare it with all the related information stored in the various layers of our memory. That is why we have such a strong urge to categorize and label things. We not only try to name them but we attach to them feelings, judgements and associations. The force of these accumulations is so strong that we react with an unquestioning conviction of "truth" or "reality." Each new reaction is in turn accumulated.

For example, imagine yourself at home. You hear a rumbling sound. You might register a mental image of the furnace in the basement, the wind, a distant motorcycle, an airplane, an intruder or perhaps even a ghost. The image will be accompanied by a feeling, such as indifference, surprise, annoyance, fear. On a physical level, all you actually experienced was a brief stimulation of your auditory mechanisms. All the rest — images, feelings, emotions — were the result of your mental conditioning (your accumulated past) replaying, readjusting and renewing itself.

The force of this conditioning is greatly magnified (and correspondingly more stressful) when it is emotionally charged. This can happen, for example, if you suspect that something you hold dear is being threatened. The more we value a particular "possession" — money, career, fame, loved ones and core beliefs like religion or personal philosophy — the greater will be our fear of losing it and the stronger will be our conditioned defensive reactions. This occurs far more frequently than we imagine because we liberally define what constitutes a "threat" and what is "ours." Someone else simply being different from you can be interpreted as a threat. People have been aggressive towards me simply because I do not eat meat.

Belief — the feeling of "I know" — is one of the subtlest and most powerful forms of conditioning. Belief may be based on personal experience or on some external authority, whether intellectual, psychological, spiritual or otherwise. As soon as you feel you know (necessarily based on the past), you are closed to the new. There is no room for change, for receiving what is fresh, because you are so full of your own knowledge. The *Tao Te Ching* advises:

"Not knowing that one knows is best;
Thinking that one knows when one does not is sickness.
Only when one becomes sick of this sickness can one be free from sickness."

We fool ourselves when we make such statements as "I believe such-and-such, but I like to keep an open mind." To *believe* means to have faith in, put trust in, accept the truth of something. This implies commitment and identification. The stronger the belief, the stronger the identification. If you identify with your belief (which is common), then when your belief is threatened, you are threatened. You defend yourself; you counterattack. This is not the sign of an open mind.

Even if we alter the contents of our belief system, we will still be caught in the process of belief itself. Any belief system, no matter how sophisticated or how high its authority, is static. It is still the past and, as such, is too rigid and cumbersome to meet the dynamic challenges of the present . No matter how much something may resemble the past, it is not the past. It is the present, needing a present response. The present moment is unique and always pregnant with possibilities of the new.

The more you know, the more difficult it is to be open to the new. You have more experience; you have more answers, explanations and convictions. Knowledge and experience, however, are no substitute for being alive to the present. Even if you have had "peak" spiritual experiences, you still have to get up each day and face life anew. An experienced driver falling asleep at the wheel will crash as surely as a novice.

In my experience of Insight Meditation, those who make the most progress are those who recognize the limitations of their belief systems and experiences. They open up to the new and quickly begin to experience real change in many areas of their lives.

Even in these cases, however, knowledge can be an impediment. As they look back with satisfaction at their achievements, the old feeling that "I know" begins to return with even greater conviction and authority than before. It is now reinforced by more profound experience. As soon as this happens, new structures of conformity are erected, choking off aliveness and blocking the pathways to change. To see with new eyes, we must be like babies. Babies do not mull over the past or project into the future.

The first step in changing is to see and feel for yourself the urgent need for radical change. Radical change is responding to each moment fully. It is unconditional and unpredictable. Setting timetables for action, imposing conditions and terms for changing, and looking outside yourself are all forms of escape from the immediacy of the moment. They create distance between you and real change. There is no such thing as "safe" change. Change is the new, which is never safe in the sense of being predictable.

Trying to change is not the same as changing. If you keep on trying but failing, it means that one part of you wants to change but another part does not. You are caught in conflict. Before you can free yourself from it, you must first recognize your predicament. Krishnamurti points out that "conflict, in which that part of the mind which wants change is trying to overcome the recalcitrant part, is called discipline, sublimation, suppression; it is also called following the ideal. An attempt is being made to build a bridge over the gap of self-contradiction . . . We pursue the ideal because it doesn't demand immediate action; the ideal is an accepted and respected postponement."

No Purpose, No Action

To open to the present, we must let go of both the past and the future. We must let go of experience, judgement, knowledge and belief; we must let go of goals and even of purpose. The catch is that there is nothing we can "do," since "doing" is itself a bridge between past and future.

We are constantly "doing" in order to "become" something else. We are not satisfied or complete the way we are. Doing and becoming give us a greater feeling of continuity and solidity. However, since we are in fact not solid (a point on which both mystics and scientists agree), we are attempting the impossible. We can never have security as we now conceive of it since everything is in a state of flux. There is nothing to which we can hold on.

If you examine your average day, you will see that you are almost always in the state of doing, which includes thinking. Your head is full of things you feel you "must" do — performing at work, looking after the children, trying to have a good time, taking care of domestic matters. Even quiet activities like reading a book or going for a walk are forms of doing. They fill the spaces in your life and conceal the lurking emptiness.

Opening to the moment is difficult because it must be purposeless. My dictionary defines *purpose* as "object to be obtained, thing intended." We cannot open to the new if we already have an object in mind, even if that object is something "reasonable" like peace or clarity. Anything that our mind can produce, it can also destroy. Our mind can neither produce nor destroy the new and unconditioned.

If there is nothing that you can do to resolve this dilemma, then do nothing. The state of not doing, however, is rare. It is unconditional. It is the complete absence of manipulation and control; it is the acceptance of yourself and your world as it is in that moment, whether this seems pleasant or unpleasant. In other words, it is the willingness to accept reality as it is. It is being rather than becoming.

When you truly give up, then you receive. Out of this stillness and emptiness can come immense transformative power. When the mind is still, there is no fear, conflict and fragmentation to consume your energies, obstruct your perception and bind you to the patterns of the past. There are instead space and energy for wisdom and creativity to manifest themselves.

You are then finally free from the past and able to respond totally to the challenge of life moment by moment. You can give one hundred percent of yourself. If you do this, then there is no more that you can do. There is no doubt, guilt or accumulation of unfinished business. Without worrying about the future, you do what is best for the future, which is total, appropriate action in the present.

Living in the present is simple, spontaneous and harmonious. If you do what you need to do, then that is the best that you can do for yourself and for your cosmos. Such action is total, and as such free of conflict. You are open to the wonder and awe of life.

IV

ACTING NON-ACTION

*"Non-action does not mean doing nothing and keeping
silent. Let everything be allowed to do what it naturally does,
so that its nature will be satisfied."*
— *CHUANG-TZU*

How can you do "non-action"? In this chapter, I will
describe, as an example of the immense transformative power of non-action, the Buddhist practice of Insight
Meditation, or Vipassana. It is not the only way of transformation, but it is the way I know. Its description will,
I hope, throw more light on the process of transformation, which is universal. The deeper we go within
ourselves, the more common ground there is.

Insight Meditation (Vipassana)

Many diverse practices go under the name of meditation. Some are little more than day-dreaming. The
majority conform to the *Oxford English Dictionary*'s
definition of *meditation* as "private devotional exercise
which consists in the continuous application of the mind
to the contemplation of some religious truth, mystery
or object of reverence, in order that the soul may
increase in love of God and holiness of life."

If you are applying your mind for a particular purpose, then it follows that you must have determined
the validity of both the purpose and the method of
application. Purpose and method are therefore your

own creation and you will find what you set out to find. This is not the new but another projection of the old — the past. The intellect cannot create or capture that which is beyond its own limitations, i.e., the enlightened, the unconditional.

All goal-oriented action, even psychotherapeutic or spiritual, is a form of "becoming." There is still distance between where you are (present) and where you want to be (future), whether this is ultimate enlightenment, truth, union with God or merely feeling secure. You are still not complete, so you must exert yourself to try to bridge that gap — to become something different. No matter how much progress you make, however, your goal is still "out there," just beyond your reach.

The process of becoming is a dualistic one. The more you seek out the Light, the holy and the attractive, the more powerful is the spectre of the Dark, of evil and of pain. Your belief may be strong, but there will always be a hint of doubt, of temptation, or of guilt. Only unconditional acceptance of "what is" can free you into the present. Otherwise, there is always something to escape or to pursue. You cannot just "be."

Some years ago, a frail-looking young woman came to my introductory Insight Meditation course. Within three to four minutes of commencing our first session of sitting meditation, she started crying loudly and painfully. Her tears flowed in a torrent, in a way I had never seen before.

Afterwards she explained that she had always been sickly. Orthodox medicine had not helped her, so she had turned to meditation. For years she had practised positive affirmation and visualization, imagining herself bathed in white, purifying light. These practices did improve her condition, but she was still incapacitated and was still looking for a solution.

That night, for the first time in her meditations, she refrained from doing anything but watching, just as I had instructed. Suddenly she vividly relived a traumatic event that had occurred when she was about two years old. She had undergone a double eye operation; she was in pain, terrified and all alone in a strange, impersonal hospital. To make matters worse, her parents never visited her in the hospital. She felt abandoned. This experience had, from her subconscious, dominated her whole life. She knew that she was not well but she did not know why. Her ideas, although intelligent and perceptive, about what she needed to do to heal herself, in fact prevented her from finding out the deeper causes of her suffering. Only when she let go of her ideas, of "doing" and of "progressing," could she truly receive.

I prefer a definition of *meditation* that is less common: "to fix one's attention upon; to observe with interest or intentness." This definition suggests immediacy, aliveness, simplicity and curiosity without the expectation of some pay-back, rather like a child looking at a snowflake for the first time.

In Insight Meditation, the object of one's attention is not some predetermined person, belief, attribute, goal or problem, but whatever is taking place in the present moment. The practice is not to control or remedy the present but to be totally immersed in it, whether it seems pleasant or unpleasant. Your awareness, therefore, is always alive and dynamic, equal to the unpredictable flow of life.

Vipassana means "to see in many ways, to see and penetrate an object thoroughly, to see with intuitive wisdom." If you can see into each moment in this way, you will see both subject and object, instead of just the object. You will see in a total way that gives rise to direct, choiceless "insight" and "wisdom" or "full knowledge." This type of insight or seeing must be distinguished from intellectual deduction and from unbridled conditioning masquerading as instinct or intuition.

Carl Jung described his own process of inner certainty in his book *Memories, Dreams, Reflections:* "When people say I am wise, or a sage, I cannot accept it . . . I am at the stream, but I do nothing. Other people are at the same stream, but most of them find they have to do something with it . . . I stand and behold, admiring what nature can do . . . The difference between most people and myself is that for me the 'dividing walls' are transparent. Others find these walls so opaque that they see nothing behind them and therefore think nothing is there. To some extent I perceive the processes going on in the background, and that gives me an inner certainty."

Insight, in the sense of total, penetrating knowledge, leads to total action. Total action is called by some "choiceless action" because there is neither doubt nor conflict. You "see" and act directly in accordance with what you see, with your whole being. Because all aspects of your being are acting in harmony, great power is generated without your seeking power. There is no gap between thought and deed; there is no accumulation, internally (for example, in suppressed emotions or in regrets) or externally, from what has been left undone. You take care of each moment as it arises so that you can face the next moment afresh and new.

A Personal Experience

A good example of the process and the power of insight occurred in my life about a year and a half after I had begun teaching meditation and Tai Chi Chuan in Toronto. A few months after I had started teaching, I was persuaded by a friend to go into the fresh seafood business with him. Very little money was coming in from my teaching and I had a family of three to support. Since the seafood business would be only part-time, it seemed "reasonable" to earn some money while I saw how my attempts at teaching developed.

I did not like the seafood business, but I regarded it as a test of my perseverance. I gave it as much attention and energy as was necessary. Over the next year or so, I learned a lot about driving large trucks on congested streets, loading and unloading thousands of pounds of fish, clams and oysters in a very short time and also dealing with the raw human side of the business. From this angle, business was considerably different from the chartered accountant's perspective.

A year later we were paying the price of success. We had grown so much that the larger businesses were beginning to take us seriously. We either had to quit or become larger to avoid being gobbled up by the corporate food chain. We chose to become larger and began to negotiate for more investment capital; we leased a fish-processing plant on Vancouver Island to ensure a continous supply.

Just then, "disaster" struck. The airline that we used ruined three shipments within the space of a month and a half by leaving them unrefrigerated in the summer heat; they then denied all liability. Prospective investors were scared off and the business collapsed. To add insult to injury, my partner sold off what assets were left and took off with the money — my money. The loss represented my entire life savings.

I felt outraged, devastated and betrayed. Although my meditation practice had kept me calm and lucid throughout the rough and tumble of the previous year, this was the last straw. My so-called friend was the immediate and primary focus for my anger.

Deeper than that, however, was a strange feeling that I had somehow been betrayed by the universe itself, by God. I had done my best — to work hard, to be honest, to be clear-minded and compassionate in all my dealings. Was this my reward? Why did this have to happen to *me* when criminals were living in luxury? I felt that I had called on my family to make great sacrifices and to trust my judgement, and they too had been betrayed. Now all the cynics could say, "I told you so. Why did you think you could be different from us?" I began to doubt my spiritual practices, even though, logically, I could see no better alternative.

After a day and a half of extreme turmoil, I decided to sit in meditation for as long as it was necessary to arrive at clarity. Years of using Insight Meditation to direct my life successfully had made me unaccustomed to and greatly disturbed by the tremendous confusion and doubt I suddenly felt. I prayed loudly (and sincerely) that if there was indeed a God, of whatever denomination or tradition, this was the time for him or her to make me a believer. An angel, a messenger or even a divine sign would suffice to convert me.

Although I needed reassurance badly, I was a sufficiently experienced meditator not to fall into the trap of creating in my mind my own saviour or "solution" just to escape my immediate uncertainty and pain. If there was a God, that being would have to speak up. I watched and waited.

Suddenly I "saw." It was not God, but my own craving for security. I realized that this craving was subtly there, right at the launching of the seafood business. Although most people would regard it as eminently "reasonable" and prudent to seek a second source of income while my teaching developed, it was clear to me that there had been a shaft of doubt within me. I did not trust totally that I should give myself to teaching even though my heart told me so. In other words, I did not totally trust my heart.

This same craving for security was also the cause of my deep feeling of betrayal. Like most people, I felt that if I did the "right" thing, then all should turn out right. When things did not appear to be turning out right, I began to question my understanding of life, even though this understanding had always made so much sense and had seemed so clear. I wanted some higher spiritual authority to come down and explain to me why things had turned out the way they had and what I had done to deserve such a fate.

As amazing as it may seem, this simple "direct seeing" or insight into my own need for security immediately vanquished all my conflicts, confusion and problems. This process was far more profound and penetrating than intellectual reasoning. I no longer needed any explanations or guidance from any authority, because everything was suddenly and choicelessly crystal clear to me. My authority was my own inner certainty.

I was able to let go of all concerns about both the past and the future. I no longer agonized over the financial losses and the possibility of legal action against me. I did not worry about where the next dollar would come from. I let go of wanting to get back at my former partner and I relinquished my anger at what seemed a wasted year and a half of my life. I suddenly had no doubt about teaching as a way of life and about my abilities as a teacher.

I simply "knew," without a doubt, that it was right for me to teach. Even though it appeared to be financial suicide, I acted on what I knew to be right for me. I poured all my time and energy into teaching. Life began to flow much more harmoniously, and my teaching grew not only in terms of number of students but in terms of my own maturity and joy. The "disaster" ultimately proved to be a rebirth. Had things gone according to my "reasonable" planning, I would probably be working full-time in the seafood business right now.

Insight, and the subsequent choiceless (without doubt) and total (without conflict) action that flowed from it, were all the result of "non-action." When I sat in meditation, I refrained from "doing" anything. I just wanted to be completely open to and observant of everything that was swirling within me. I did not attempt to sort it out, because that would have made my head spin with even more speculation and reasoning. I did nothing but open myself to everything that was happening, without judging, suppressing or manipulating. My meditation was finally brought to an end by someone knocking at the door. To my surprise, two and a half hours had passed; it had seemed like minutes.

To me, non-action is the same as total action. Non-action is not the lack of activity but the lack of disharmonious activity. It is a response that arises out of direct, choiceless insight into what is needed in that moment, not out of the ego's need for expansion or security. It is not the projection of beliefs, desires or expectations; it is based not on probability but on direct knowing.

When you practise non-action, you can be as versatile as water. You can be absolutely still or you can surge powerfully forward; you can retreat or advance with equal facility; you can flow over, around or through obstacles. Your response is then governed not by your habitual patterns of behaviour (the past) but by what is necessary in each moment. It is therefore appropriate, harmonious and without conflict. It is total.

We can sometimes observe non-action or total action in exceptional athletes. They seem calm, even-keeled and perhaps even strangely distant. Their movements tend to be flowing, unhurried and effortless, as if they have all the time in the world. Yet they are capable not only of generating immense speed and power but of adapting to every situation and every change in their opponents' strategy. Their ego does not get in the way of what they have to do; they can concentrate totally on the business at hand. Simplicity, humility and sensitivity are transformed into intelligent power. Total action in our everyday life is an even rarer and greater achievement than in the limited confines of a sport. It is, nevertheless, something we must all attempt.

Total action should not be confused with action fuelled by powerful belief or conviction, whether religious or otherwise. They are often mistaken for the same thing, because, on the surface, they may appear very similar. Both involve concentration, energy, power and, in many cases, result in great achievement. Whereas, however, non-action or total action is characterized by softness and flexibility, belief generates rigidity and hardness. What is hard cannot bend. When hardness comes up against something that is also hard, there is collision and breakage. What is hard will ultimately be overcome by what is soft. There is a saying in Tai Chi Chuan that "Four ounces can deflect a thousand pounds."

Instructions for Sitting Meditation

The heart of Insight Meditation practice is sitting meditation. Sitting quietly, with a minimum of external distraction, you can begin to listen to the internal sounds and to observe the varied activity within. You can begin to look at the looker. In time, you will be able to meditate even when engaged in an activity. Sitting meditation, though, is a convenient starting point and a way of creating immediate space and perspective in your life. Albert Einstein, in a letter to Queen Elizabeth of Belgium, wrote: "Perhaps, some day, solitude will come to be properly recognized and appreciated as the teacher of personality. The Orientals have long known this. The individual who has experienced solitude will not easily become a victim of mass suggestion."

Clear Intention

The first requirement for meditation, as with any other activity, is what the Buddhists call "clear comprehension of purpose." (The "purpose" in Vipassana is not the attainment of a particular state but simply to be aware and open in the present moment.) Before you begin, initially and at the commencement of each session, ask yourself if you really see the necessity of meditating, if you really want to meditate.

If the answer is yes, then do it. If the answer is yes, but . . . then you are in conflict; you are not really clear; you will find excuses for procrastination and avoidance. If the answer is no, then do whatever it is you want to do. Clarity of purpose is your priority.

In the long run, we cannot avoid dealing with ourselves. Sooner or later, in spite of our ego's desire to feel in control, life's painful lessons will bring us all back to the need for the resolution of our conflicts, to the need for real change. Sooner resolution is better than later, because the destructive energies inside us accumulate. If they reach the point of explosion or disintegration, it may be too late. The conflict and pain are already there. Meditation does not create them but only brings them to consciousness so that we can release them.

Time and Place

If you have clarity regarding meditation, then you need to arrange a suitable time and place. It is best (though not essential) to reserve a fixed time in your daily schedule. Many people find that first thing in the morning is the most convenient. The mind tends to be quieter, the body is refreshed by sleep, and it is an excellent way to start the day. Excuses like "I am not a morning person" or "I need so many hours of sleep" are usually just that — excuses. Heavy meals tend to make you drowsy, so wait a while after eating before meditating. Each person tends to have a daily pattern of times of high or low energy. During low-energy periods, it is more difficult to pay attention and drowsiness is more likely.

I suggest timing the period of meditation. (If your timing device is noisy, put it under a pillow to muffle the sound.) Start with about twenty minutes of meditation and gradually work up to about an hour. These periods are merely suggestions. Longer sittings do not necessarily mean better-quality sittings; they just give you more time during which to experience yourself and your patterns. I find that if meditators do not make a commitment to a specific period of meditation but rather sit as long as it feels "good," then they are usually deepening the basic pattern of pleasure/pain. If you never stay to investigate discomfort, you always have to run away from it. It will always control you.

Any quiet space is suitable for Insight Meditation. Absolute silence is not essential, because the mind, although concentrated, is at the same time open and receptive. If there are sounds, they are watched as they rise and fall. Attempts to resist or exclude sound usually result in further mental discomfort. Good ventilation helps. Light should be subdued and the room temperature moderate. It is a good idea to keep a light shawl or sweater nearby as sometimes you may experience changes in body temperature. Wear loose clothing, especially around the stomach area.

Body Posture

The body should be relaxed during meditation. If you find you are not relaxed, it may help to do some gentle breathing and stretching exercises before you begin. For example, as you inhale deeply into the abdomen, let your arms rise up sideways, palms up as if gathering energy. Continue until they meet above your head. As you exhale, let them slowly descend in front of you, relaxing the wrists, the elbows and finally the shoulders. Let the breath "melt" your body from the head to the feet. Repeat until you feel more relaxed and are breathing more deeply. You can loosen up further by rotating your neck, arms and waist.

To meditate, you may sit either in a chair or cross-legged on a cushion. If you sit on a chair, make sure your feet are flat on the ground and that you are not leaning against the chair back. A padded seat helps. If you prefer a cushion, choose a firm one that will raise you approximately six inches off the ground. Sit with your legs folded in front of your body, one in front of the other, in such a way that the outsides of your lower legs are resting on the ground. If your legs are not flexible enough to do this, you can wedge flat pillows underneath your knees to support you. Those with greater flexibility may sit, without a cushion, in the lotus or half-lotus position.

I am often asked why one should sit cross-legged rather than in a chair. Some people feel that this position is alien to Westerners. Although it is not necessary to sit cross-legged, I recommend it because, once you are accustomed to it, your body is far more stable. The posture also facilitates the movement of energy around your body.

If the cross-legged posture causes you discomfort initially, you can use this as a valuable opportunity to observe the process of discomfort and pain. The duality of pleasure and pain rules our lives. It is something we must all face, sooner or later, during self-enquiry. As incredible as it may seem at first, the movement towards comfort and away from discomfort is not a "natural" inevitability but is another conditioning pattern from which you must free yourself. If you remain within the pattern, you are not open to the new. Avoidance of pain is what keeps it trapped inside us. If you sit for long enough in a comfortable chair, you will also experience discomfort. It is just a question of how long you take to get to the point of discomfort.

Once you are seated and ready to begin meditating, check your body once again. Your upper body should be upright but relaxed, with chest and shoulders down. Tilt your head down slightly, with the chin tucked in. The lower part of your body is also relaxed, but solidly supported by the ground, the chair seat or by firm cushions, so that it does not tilt or wobble.

There are many variations in hand positions, but here are the basic and simple ones. Hands may be placed in your lap, one above the other, palms up with the thumbs touching. They may rest, palms down or up, on the knees. Initially, choose the position that feels most comfortable.

Some people find it helpful to do a brief progressive relaxation exercise before the meditation *per se*. This practice consists of mentally scanning the whole body, checking it for tension and letting go of any that is found. You can start at the feet and move up to the calves, knees and thighs. Next, scan the buttocks, the lower back, the shoulders and then down the arms into the hands. Continue up the back of the neck, over the top of the head, down the face, throat, chest, and finally to the abdomen. It may help to think of your tissues melting or dissolving. Keep on letting go and opening up, both body and mind, allowing yourself just to be.

The Mind

To start your practice of Insight Meditation, bring your attention to the physical sensations caused by the rising and falling of your breath. You need give only what is called "bare attention" to your breathing without any visualization, verbalization, regulation, counting or categorization. These are unnecessary mental overlays that obscure the simple awareness of the physical sense of touch (the rising and falling of the stomach or chest caused by breathing).

You may find that within a matter of seconds your attention has moved elsewhere. You may be thinking of what you did yesterday or what you will do tomorrow; you may be making mental "to do" lists. You may find yourself distracted by noise, by temperature or by a variety of bodily sensations. You may start thinking about meditation itself. You may wonder if you are doing it correctly or you may feel self-conscious. You may feel bored, restless, frustrated, fearful, even angry. You may not even be aware that your attention has wandered and that you are now thinking about your breathing rather than just feeling it.

One meditator told me that she had no problem meditating since her mind was always quiet and empty. Finding this rather unusual, I enquired further and discovered that she imagined her mind to be a huge movie screen and whenever there were any thoughts, she would run them off the screen, like movie credits, into a huge garbage bin at the bottom of the screen. Employing the mind is just another form of control. It is action that inevitably provokes reaction — the restless mind. Allowing emptiness to arise spontaneously is a completely natural process.

As soon as you become aware that your attention has wandered from the mere physical sensations of breathing, acknowledge where your attention is, let go, and gently start over with the breath. By acknowledging where and how the mind has strayed, you are also learning about its patterns and its concerns. You are cultivating insight. For example, if you notice that your mind constantly worries during meditation, then it is likely that it also worries all day long. As you continue your meditation practice, you will learn more about the precise mechanisms and causes of your particular worrying process. You will also notice it more quickly when it occurs in your everyday life.

Letting go and starting over are entirely different from forcing the mind back through willpower. Force often provokes reaction and deepens conflict — between the controller and the controlled, the good and the bad. There is an ongoing struggle to overcome by force; there is often frustration.

Starting over is one of the most valuable lessons that you can learn, since every moment of your life is always new, always different. You must let go of the past in order to start afresh. By letting go and starting over, you forgive yourself and create new beginnings; you also cultivate patience, compassion and mental equilibrium.

You may find sometimes during your meditation practice that you are experiencing deep peace and stillness, joy, or flashes of insight into your life. Be aware and receptive to whatever is happening, but do not interfere. Do not try to prolong the experience or to make "sense" of it. When it is over, do not try to recreate it, since that would be moving away from being, back into the process of becoming — moving from here to there, now to then. In the practice of Insight Meditation, you neither push away the unpleasant nor seek to hold on to the pleasant. Thus, you avoid attachment.

Occasionally, it may seem impossible to bring your mind back to your breathing, because something is calling (or screaming) for your attention. It may be pain in the body or some strong emotion like anger or fear; it may be an image or a memory of some incident in your life; it may be an unusual or mystical experience.

At such times, since you have little choice, make whatever is happening the object of your meditation. As with the breath, however, do not interfere, judge or enter into an internal discussion. Just allow and observe, even if you are scared. In this way, your meditation will become more flowing and dynamic, opening you to the possibility of the new, the unknown, and to real transformation.

It is important to maintain continuity in your meditation practice, during each session and as part of your daily routine. Insight Meditation is a commitment to ongoing awareness; it is a journey of discovery. It is not dependent on progress, results or mood swings.

During your meditation practice, open yourself totally to being with yourself in the moment. When you start exercising discrimination and judgement about what is happening, you immediately move from the unconditional back to the conditional, back to the closed cycle of duality. It is extremely easy to find a reason not to meditate, because a strong part of your being is scared and threatened by self-discovery. The "I" does not want to surrender its power and control.

I see the practice of Vipassana as creating space within the present moment. We normally do not experience this space because it is immediately filled with our ideas and knowledge. The more you allow yourself to be in the moment, the more space you create for yourself — to be free from the compulsions of past patterns and to look into the causes and mechanisms of those patterns, no matter how insignificant they may seem at first.

For example, one of my students was having difficulty with certain seemingly simple Tai Chi Chuan movements. Her unhesitating explanation was that she was not a "physical" person and maybe Tai Chi was not for her. One night as I watched her I saw her mental attitudes clearly manifesting themselves in her physical movements. I pointed out that she seemed anxious about moving and was hurrying to put her foot back on the ground. Because she was trying to step down before she was properly balanced, she became even more unbalanced and was almost stumbling forward.

Her eyes lit up with instant recognition. She suddenly realized that these simple physical movements precisely reflected a deeply held but hitherto unquestioned attitude to life. Whenever there was any space in her life that was not filled with activity, she would rush to find something to fill it because she could not stand the uncertainty and the emptiness. Since this activity was driven by anxiety rather than by consideration of what was appropriate in the circumstances, it usually added further complication and stress to her life. This insight led to an immediate improvement not only in her Tai Chi but also in her ability to handle her anxiety and her life in general.

As you continue to practise Insight Meditation, your mind will become quiet and your wisdom and compassion will grow. These processes do not always or necessarily manifest themselves during sitting meditation. They may become manifest only after you have confronted and released your personal demons.

Many people find that, almost imperceptibly, they are seeing and doing things differently in their daily lives. The quality of their lives changes in subtle but profound ways. Others experience far more dramatic change, sometimes involving a change of partner or career. Often a person's face or even body shape can alter dramatically; as the mind becomes more natural, balanced and alive, the body reflects these changes.

All these changes are the result of opening yourself to the new, to the other. The more you open yourself, the more you can receive and the more you can give. The more you accept the unknown and the risky, the less you have to fear. Instead of life being a journey towards death, it becomes a timeless and ever-fresh moment of exploration, challenge and wonder. By accepting death, you become more alive.

Auxiliary Meditation Exercises

Strictly speaking, Insight Meditation does not need auxiliary exercises. If you practise Vipassana skilfully, you will have insight into what needs doing and how to do it. Direct insight (as opposed to intellectual knowledge) can be far more profound than "expert" opinion, which is always second-hand. Even if you need to consult specialists for technical expertise and knowledge, your own inner knowing (insight) will remain your main guide. It is never lacking.

What may be lacking, however, is balance in the way you practise your meditation. It is easy to latch onto one or another aspect of the practice and forget the rest, especially if you do not have a teacher or experienced spiritual friend to alert you to your oversight. The following exercises help restore balance to your practice.

Concentration (Samatha)

Sometimes the mind becomes so passive that it cannot focus. Concentration (Samatha) meditation techniques help to focus the mind. The ultimate goal of Samatha meditation is the complete unification of the mind with its object, to the exclusion of all else. It is in essence quite different from Vipassana, wherein the mind remains open and accommodating. In some schools of Buddhism, Samatha is regarded as a preliminary stage in the attainment of Vipassana.

Counting the breath is a common concentration technique. Regarding each inhalation-exhalation as "one," count from one to five. Repeat the one-to-five count until your mind is sufficiently alert and focused, then return to the basic Vipassana practice of just feeling the physical sensations of the breath.

Another simple concentration technique is "following the breath," paying close attention to three physical points during each inhalation and exhalation. On the inhalation, feel the breath in the nose, at the centre of the chest and then at the navel. On the exhalation, feel the breath first at the navel, then at the chest and, finally, at the nose. Repeat until basic concentration is established, then return to Vipassana.

Meditation on Universal Love and Benevolence (Metta)

In Buddhism, skilful spiritual practice leads to the development of the Twin Virtues, Wisdom (Panna) and Compassion (Karuna). Wisdom is the Head, the intellect. Compassion includes the loving qualities of the Heart — love, tenderness and openness. Since Insight Meditation may be classified as a Wisdom practice, it is prudent to check that the Heart is not being neglected.

Metta Meditation is a guided meditation that focuses on the Heart. Bring your attention to the spiritual heart centre, in the middle of the chest, trying to feel the expansion and contraction caused by the breath. Next, try to feel warm and loving energy there. Once you can feel it, enable it to radiate throughout the whole body. If you cannot do this, then be aware of what you do feel — tightness, coldness, or whatever. This, too, is valuable information concerning your internal state.

Having accumulated loving feelings, direct them to yourself, forgiving yourself for all mistakes and wrongdoings. The past is past and cannot be relived. Let go of self-criticism and self-hatred. Give yourself the opportunity to make a fresh start in the present moment.

Having given love to yourself, now direct it to those closest to you: your spouse, partner, children, parents, siblings, intimate friends. Forgive them for any hurt that they may have caused you; feel the love and affection they have given you; mentally embrace them. Let go of any ill-feeling you may be harbouring towards them.

Next, forgive those you hate or fear and those who have hurt you, either intentionally or unintentionally. Realize that they are caught in their patterns of conditioning as much as you are in yours. Let go of all negative emotions; remember that these are stored in your body and psyche, and they damage you much more than the object of your negativity. You cannot free yourself if you are attached to hatred. You become hatred.

Finally, extend your loving compassion in ever-increasing circles to friends, acquaintances, your community, your country, the whole of humanity and then to all living beings. Take as much time as you feel is necessary to complete each section of this meditation, to embrace these larger circles. At the conclusion of your Metta meditation, return to your basic Vipassana practice of just watching the breath.

Who Am I?

The "I" — the ego or sense of personal self — is extremely confusing. On the one hand, it seems solid. We feel ourselves to be substantial; society treats us as solid, separate entities; psychological experts talk about building self-esteem so that the ego/self can feel solid and function effectively in the world. On the other hand, however, if we look for this entity, it cannot be found as something substantial. Very little is known about the real nature of the "I," even though we act as "I" most of the time. For this reason, "I" has been described in this book as a huge blind-spot in our consciousness.

Vipassana helps you to look behind the apparent solidity of everyday reality. What looks solid usually turns out to be a process or a series of interlocking processes. Although this may be quite disturbing at first, it helps to make much more sense of the seeming chaos that is life. As Jung explained, "I perceive the processes going on in the background, and that gives me an inner certainty."

If you understand the nature of your ego, it can function as a highly effective tool without the distortion of attachment or compulsion. This is rather different from developing a strong sense of ego (often called self-esteem). No matter how strong and confident the ego feels at any given time, it is living in a world of illusion. By its very nature, it is not substantial and therefore can never feel solid and secure enough. It comes into being only with the process of thought. If "I" has no memory, it cannot exist.

Sometimes in meditation, you may find it impossible to disentangle yourself from your ego, even with all the above insights. You may find yourself overwhelmed by the intensity of the ego: "I hate," "I am mad, hurt," "My body hurts," "I am afraid, terrified," "I deserve," "I am depressed, frustrated," "I have great power." One of the simplest and most profound antidotes to this identification is to continue asking yourself the question, "Who am I?" Whatever answer your intellect provides, press on with "Who am I?" By doing this, you can enquire into the very essence of your being.

For example, you may start with the obvious identification: the body. Are you the limbs, the trunk, the organs, the bones, the head, the brains, the physical sensations, the emotions, the feelings, the thinking processes? Are you any of the roles that you play — familial, sexual, professional, racial, religious, intellectual or spiritual?

Even if you never come up with a definitive intellectual answer to this question, you can at least discover the many things that you are not. The more you let go of your identification with what you are not, the closer you naturally come to what you really are.

Slow Walking Meditation

Walking meditation introduces both simple conscious activity and physical movement into your meditation practice. It helps you to become more aware of your body and to begin applying your mindfulness practice in daily life.

Walking requires very little thinking as it is usually one of our earliest major physical accomplishments. Because it is so simple and because it plays such an important part in our lives, it is an ideal object for our attention.

Start off in a standing posture with your knees slightly bent and your torso erect but relaxed. Look straight ahead. As with sitting meditation, bring your attention to your breathing and just stand without moving, feeling solidly supported by the ground.

As you become aware of the intention to move, mindfully shift the weight to one leg and lift the other. Be conscious of the first phase of walking, which is "lifting." The second stage of walking is "extending," as you move your foot forward and lightly touch the heel to the ground. Now be aware of the final stage, touching, as you commit your weight to your forward leg. As the front foot completes touching, the back foot will commence lifting. As you walk, continue to distinguish these three stages of walking.

It may help to use the Tai Chi method of breathing, which is to inhale as you lift your foot and exhale as you place it on the ground. Breathe into the lower stomach area, just below the navel; the chest and shoulders sink down. Keep your upper body relaxed and upright, with your knees bent at all times, especially when you are standing on one leg. Walk as slowly and mindfully as you can without losing your balance.

As with sitting meditation, whenever your attention wanders, acknowledge where it is, let go and gently bring it back to the awareness of the three phases of "just walking." Learn to give your attention to only one thing at a time.

At times your attention may be drawn to some particular part of the body or aspect of the walking movement. For example, you may notice your body leaning to one side, tensions in certain parts of your body, irregularity in your breathing, slouching, weight being placed either on the inside or outside of your foot, imbalance as you stand on one leg, a sensation of falling forward as you step, a tendency to look around or to scratch yourself. Notice not only the physical details of your tendencies but also the attitudes and emotions connected with them. For example, hunching your shoulders forward might be a way of trying to protect yourself from the uncertainties of life or, for some women, a way of hiding the breasts; reluctance to physically commit your weight may reflect a fear of commitment in general; a left-right imbalance usually signifies an imbalance between female and male energies or unresolved conflicts with mother or father.

Many chronic postural or other health problems can be remedied by simple insight. For example, because many seniors are anxious about falling, they tend to hunch forward to look at the ground and to take quick, shuffling steps. The hunching constricts the breathing, curves the spine and causes unnecessary tension and makes them lurch forward as they step, increasing the likelihood of falling.

Insight Meditation can help not only in reducing the anxiety associated with walking but in improving the actual mechanisms of walking. If you walk with an upright posture and breathe properly, tension in the body and the tendency to lurch forward are decreased. If you touch the heel down first before committing your weight (as in slow, meditative walking), you will reduce the likelihood of slipping.

Obstacles to the Practice

The Buddha listed Five Hindrances to clear understanding and progress in meditation (they apply to all endeavours): desire for sensations; ill-will, hatred or anger; sloth and torpor; restlessness and worry; and sceptical doubt.

Desire for sensations includes the physical senses as well as the "passions" such as envy, jealousy, possessiveness, pride, arrogance and conceit. When we cite boredom as an excuse for inaction, it is usually because we desire sensation. We want something stimulating, exciting, pleasurable. If something pleasant is not available, we often take the unpleasant in preference to nothing. In therapy and meditation, having a traumatic problem to work on is often engrossing and satisfying. We all know people who get satisfaction out of a good fight.

Our attention span and our ability to do without constant stimulation seem to be decreasing. Actors, entertainers and media people all work to make an immediate impression, to arrest our attention, to keep us stimulated and to sum up complicated issues in few words. As we become accustomed to this sort of communication, we find it increasingly difficult to listen and to make space for sensitivity. At the end of a one-hour lecture, during which I had tried mightily to sum up the contents of this book, a member of the audience complained that while my ideas were interesting, she still had not learnt the secret of integrating body and mind! She wanted a definite concept and technique that yielded immediate results.

Though we think of ourselves as sharp and on the cutting edge of what is happening, we are actually becoming duller and more insensitive. We need more and more extreme forms of stimulation in order to feel anything. That is why sex, violence and drug abuse are so common in our culture and are becoming more extreme. Many of us go to horror films for relaxation.

Looking to spirituality for stimulation is relatively healthy, but in the end it is the same process. If we cannot just "be," we must constantly "do" and "become" in order to fill up our emptiness and cover over our inadequacies. So we look for something out of the ordinary, dramatic, inspiring, uplifting. In doing so, we presume that spirituality is not within the ordinary and is not here and now.

When my children cite boredom as an excuse, I point out that nothing is intrinsically boring. Boredom arises in the individual; it is the individual that is boring at that moment. Boredom is irrelevant. If the action needs to be done, do it. If not, don't do it.

Most of us would condemn ill-will, hatred and anger. We hate these emotions in other people, yet we find so many reasons for excusing them in ourselves. "I am justified because I have been wronged," "I had a stressful day," "I am fighting for a noble cause," "My anger is righteous/constructive."

As with desire for sensations, apply your meditation practice. Watch how anger arises, manifests itself and falls away. Do not identify with it or become attached to it; do not justify it. See that anger is actually an obstruction to effective action since it distorts your perception and causes divisiveness, hurt and guilt. If you are already angry, let it go. It is not healthy to keep anger stored inside you, no matter how righteous you think it is. Often it is not the outburst of anger that causes problems, but the aftermath — the guilt, the hurt and the justifications.

The third hindrance is sloth, torpor. This is the attitude that you should not do anything that is not absolutely necessary. Let sleeping dogs lie and hope all will be well. In Insight Meditation practice, it is true that self-enquiry can bring painful memories and even physical pain to your consciousness. Meditation, however, does not create that pain. The pain is already there, dangerously suppressed inside your body and influencing your actions in subconscious, destructive ways.

If you are not conscious of your pain and of what needs to be remedied, you cannot take remedial action. If there is nothing wrong with you, then you have nothing to lose through self-enquiry. If there is something amiss, you do not benefit by ignoring it. All big problems start as little ones.

The hindrances of restlessness and worry prevent the development of a calm and insightful mind. Worrying about the future does not make the future safer or better. It may in fact make it worse, since it distracts you from what you need to do now. Again, clear comprehension of purpose is helpful. Determine your best course of action for the future and then implement it step by step. If it is not yet time to take the first step, turn your attention to the challenge of the present moment.

Sceptical doubt is perhaps the most serious of the hindrances. Dhiravamsa explains: "The moment one sees and understands, doubt disappears completely . . . It is good to begin with doubts and reservations . . . Such doubt encourages investigation of the facts and a search for the truth underlying them. When one perceives reality through one's own investigation, doubt is removed . . . On the other hand, the hindrance of Sceptical Doubt implies an innate bias which prevents investigation, a form of doubt which does not want to know. If this condition is very strong, little can be done until the impermanence of life has wrought its inevitable changes, and opportunity [to continue the practice] knocks once more."

Sceptical doubt can arise at any stage of your meditation practice. It is what prevents most of us from seeing the need for real change in the first place. It is a form of doubt that, even under the guise of abundant knowledge and open-mindedness, does not want to know. I find that many people who attend my introductory courses on meditation are not searching for truth so much as for something to reinforce or fine-tune what they already believe.

For those who do embark on the practice of meditation, sceptical doubt might next arise if there are no (or not enough) positive "results" to reassure them that they have done the correct thing. This is not unreasonable, but too often meditators blame the practice as not being right for them without having truly opened themselves to it. Others soon come across what they need to work on, but finding it unpleasant, cite that as a reason why Insight Meditation is not suitable for them.

I point out to these people that since there is no "doing" in Insight Meditation, and that the practice is simply being with yourself, what they do not like is not the thing they call meditation, but themselves. If you do not like being with yourself, that is a serious matter, which no amount of activity can ever successfully hide. To like being with yourself, you must first understand why you do not, which is the purpose of Insight Meditation.

Sceptical doubt plagues even those meditators who have been "successful," in the sense of having experienced positive and profound changes in their lives through meditation. As you continue the practice of Insight Meditation, you go deeper into yourself. The rewards are greater, but so are the fears. The ego or "I" sees its control shrinking. It tries to reclaim its territory through subtle subterfuges. The more you truly know yourself, however, the less you can fool yourself.

Eventually, the experienced meditator approaches a sort of "door" to the unknown. On this side of the door is the known, which for many people is quite painful. On the other side of the door is the promise of things too great even to imagine. It is surprising how many people, even though they may be in great pain and even though they may already have experienced the process of real change, fall back in fear from that doorway.

The adage "The devil you know is better than the devil you don't know" arises from a very deep part of the human psyche. No matter how great your experience of suffering, it has its limitations and its dimensions. It is within the realm of the known, and as such you can exercise some control over it, or think you can. When you approach the unknown, on the other hand, you lose your power to control. There are no familiar landmarks of experience; your " I" feels lost and in danger of extinction. This is actually the best time for a spiritual breakthrough — for loosening the stranglehold of the "I."

At such times in the practice, I advise doing what you always have to do — which is to take one step at a time. The practice releases you from great fears in the same way that it releases you from lesser fears. Instead of focusing on the content of your fears, look at the process of fear itself. Allow it and watch it as it rises and as it falls away. See it for what it is — a transitory process. Everything in the universe is subject to change, without exception.

According to the Buddhist scriptures, as you progress in the practice of Vipassana meditation, you will see for yourself the three characteristics of all phenomenal existence: impermanence, impersonality (lack of a real self) and suffering. We suffer because we are attached to and continually promoting the illusion of ourselves as a permanent and substantial entity, when in reality we are not. The closer we look, the less we will see. Some fear this as extinction; others rejoice in it as liberation and a return to our true source.

V

PRACTICAL SPIRITUALITY

*"To achieve Buddhahood, there is no need for cultivation.
Just carry on an ordinary task without any attachment.
Release your bowels and urine, wear your clothes, eat your
meals. When you are tired, lie down. The fool will laugh at
you, but the wise man will understand."*
— CH'AN (ZEN) MASTER LIN-CHI

*"Life in the world and life in the spirit are not incompatible.
Work, or action, is not contrary to the knowledge of God, but
indeed, if performed without attachment, is a means to it. On
the other hand, renunciation is renunciation of the ego,
of selfishness — not of life."*
— THE UPANISHADS

I see spirituality not only as compatible with ordinary
life but also as an indispensable ingredient. Without
spirituality, we inflict a great deal of senseless suffering and brutality on ourselves and others, because we
act in almost total ignorance of our true nature. Not
surprisingly, many feel life to be crushingly senseless
and hopeless.

Popular religion has for centuries provided hope
and various belief systems (often "divine revelations")
that try to explain the seeming futility of life. Although
religion in this sense is seen as a refuge from the world,
secular belief systems like communism and capitalism
can also fulfil the same role. They too can provide

comfort, hope, an analysis of past mistakes and a vision of the future.

I do not regard any belief system as spirituality because belief is rigid and divisive. Belief pertains to the past; it is not living. Belief by its very nature is also dualistic. It perpetuates strife and conflict because as soon as there is a believer, there is also a non-believer — God/the Devil, the saved/the damned, East/West, North/South, left/right.

Spirituality, to me, is the living present. It is the process of becoming whole. You can become whole only by first seeing for yourself how and why you are not whole and then letting go of what keeps you unwhole. This direct insight into yourself, and into life in general, is quite a different process from that of belief. Insight does not create fragments and division. On the contrary, it allows you to recognize and integrate the oneness behind your apparent separateness.

Because Insight Meditation is simple and formless, it can be applied to any situation, at any depth of your being. Insight is not a thing, it is a way. If you have learnt that way, then you can have a direct understanding of matters that may take years or decades of scientific research to substantiate. You simply know and you act in accordance with that knowing. Although this may sound like megalomania to some, insight is not concerned with protecting or inflating the ego.

What follows are some suggestions (some traditional, some not) about how you can start applying Insight Meditation in everyday life situations.

Formal Meditation Practice

Like a two-way radio, you cannot receive when you are broadcasting. One of the simplest and most immediate ways of creating the space to receive is the practice of sitting meditation, as described in the previous chapter. It is not just another form of doing but an opportunity to be, to look and to listen. I suggest at least twenty minutes a day. Longer or more frequent sessions would be a bonus.

Group meditation, say once a week, creates another type of space. It not only gives some focus and impetus to your week, but it allows you to see yourself reflected in other people. On a more superficial level, you may recognize your behavioural patterns in others; you can see yourself through another's eyes. At a deeper level, you may recognize universal issues that transcend the superficial differences between individual behavioural patterns and beliefs.

Groups also provide an opportunity for you to apply your meditation practice in relationships. All life is relationship. Even if you shut yourself in a room, you are still in relationship — although a constricted one — with life. Being part of a group, you are making a commitment to something outside yourself. There is much to be learnt about the arts of simply listening (without judgement) and speaking (from the heart). We rarely do this and, consequently, add to our own and others' confusion and conflicts.

The more you trust yourself, the more you trust others, and vice versa. In time, you can learn to be open and loving to others without wanting or needing anything from them. You truly accept them as they are, even if you do not understand or agree with their actions or words. When necessary, you can relate on the level of our underlying oneness and beingness.

Slowing Down and Making Space
In the sitting practice of Insight Meditation, there is absolutely no "doing." This quiet space of no-doing makes easier the recognition of those inner processes of which you are normally unaware. Yet Vipassana is much more than sitting in solitude. It is a way of being. It is living with increased awareness every moment of your life.

You can start to bring awareness into your everyday activities by slowing down and making space for it. Do just one thing at a time, mindfully (it cannot actually be otherwise) and stop filling the spaces in your life with superfluous activity.

Planning your life according to priorities or a sequence of events is desirable. But you can do only one thing at a time. If you determine what that is, just do it and let go of the rest. There is nothing more you can do. Feeling pressured by all the things you think you "ought" to do is an unnecessary burden that you yourself create. That involves psychological rather than chronological time.

If there is nothing to do, then do nothing. Refrain from activity for its own sake. Listening to the radio, watching television or reading are all worthwhile pursuits, but often we use them to fill the emptiness in our lives. If we do not allow ourselves to explore or understand emptiness and aloneness, then we must always run away from them. Many people remain in miserable relationships simply because they cannot bear the thought of being alone.

Use the space that you create to pay closer attention to your daily activities. It is best to start out with simple physical activities. Walking to the bus or the subway, for example, might seem a nuisance to you because it takes so much precious time out of your day and because you have to do it in all kinds of weather. You might even try to eliminate the inconvenience by buying yourself a car (although this might in turn create a financial inconvenience).

Paying mindful attention to the process of walking brings you back to the present. Thinking ahead and worrying will not make the bus come faster or get work done at your workplace. As you begin to make more space for yourself just to be, you will become more aware of yourself (your physical and mental state) and of the things and people that surround you. They will become more alive to you and your insight will deepen. You will realize that cold and rainy is not terrible, it just is — cold and rainy. As you become more spacious and accepting, there will be less to complain about and less to "rectify." You might even save yourself the added burden of a car loan!

Eventually, you will be able to maintain your awareness and concentration even when complex and intense activity is swirling around you. You will be able to establish a calm and aware "centre" within yourself, independent of what is happening externally.

Applying the Four Aspects of Mindfulness

Each activity arises from and is a precise reflection of yourself. As such, it has more to teach you about your life than books, lectures or sermons. Since all parts are connected, continued mindfulness will increase your insight into yourself, in terms of both depth of being and breadth of experience.

The Buddha described four basic foundations or aspects of mindfulness to which you can direct your attention during your daily activities: the body (physical sensations, posture); feelings (pleasant, unpleasant, indifferent); states of mind or moods; and mind-objects (the contents of thought). Mindfulness of the body is the simplest because the body is tangible. Paying attention to the sensations of breathing during sitting meditation is an example of body mindfulness. A more generalized form of body mindfulness that you can use during the course of your day is mindfulness of body posture. Make a mental note every time you change your basic body posture — lying, sitting, standing or walking. In looking at the body this way, you will become less attached and identified with it, and you will learn to use your body more efficiently.

Repetitive physical tasks are ideal subjects for body mindfulness since the mind is not too engrossed in thinking as you perform them. Instead of blanking out your mind to cope with the apparent tedium, you can actually make the mind more alive by paying attention to every detail. Let the body and mind work efficiently and in harmony. You will do a better job, and as you pay full attention to each moment you will cease checking the clock. Time will cease to drag.

At home, many activities are suitable for body mindfulness: ironing, washing dishes, mowing the lawn, dusting, polishing, vacuuming, painting. Look for the most efficient way to do the job. Check your posture and your breathing; make sure that no part of your body is tense and that all parts are working in harmony, without resistance. With body awareness, many "chores" can be transformed into health-enhancing physical workouts.

You can also practise mindfulness of feelings, state of mind and mind-objects in connection with any of these tasks. As in sitting meditation, the psychological patterns that you notice during your simple mindfulness practice are quite often influential patterns in your life in general. For example, some people actually like repetitive housework because it relaxes them and they can lose themselves in the activity. Mindfulness may reveal the state of mind to be lethargic and the mind-objects to be general or particular fantasies or day-dreaming. This is not "bad" as such, but it merits attention because it may reflect a more general attitude to life. This could be a significant factor when the situation is more meaningful, for example, if decisive action is required at work or to save a relationship.

Mindfulness is especially important when the activity in question generates conflict and stress. People who dislike domestic chores often treat them as a "necessary evil" and do not question them at a deeper level. Since these tasks are performed regularly, however, such people are in effect fighting with themselves regularly.

Mindfulness of the body often reveals tension as you "steel" yourself to perform your "chore." Mindfulness of feelings might reveal unpleasantness; the state of mind might reflect resentment, which easily ignites into irritation and anger.

Mindfulness of mental objects might reveal a whole range of assumptions and ideas that cause the resentment. Domestic matters may be judged "boring" (lacking stimulation), "menial" (degrading, servile) or "women's work," which is likely to cause resentment in both men and women. They are, in fact, none of these things. These assumptions are your own creations and as such you can let go of them. Come back to present reality; establish clarity of purpose and of method. If a given activity is necessary, then do it with totality. If it isn't necessary, don't do it.

Paying someone else to perform the tasks you regard as menial is not the solution that it may seem initially. Often this just transfers the stigma of housework to someone else.

Our domestic life merits our utmost attention, for it consumes a substantial amount of our time and energy. What's more, it concerns our home, our private refuge. If we cannot literally and figuratively keep our own house in order, we have no right to tell other people how to run theirs.

The stigma of domesticity is often subconsciously extended to the raising of children. Society extols the virtue of the family but does not reward the homemakers. Raising a family is seen by many men and women as an inferior role or function. As individuals, we like the idea of having children but often have neither the time nor inclination to raise them.

The children often pay the price for our confusion. Many people find themselves working full-time just to pay someone else to do their parenting for them! Since parenting is such an inexact undertaking and involves such powerful, unpredictable and long-term forces, getting someone to do the job, in some cases, would seem an unnecessary and potentially damaging complication of life.

Much of the confusion and conflict regarding family life stems from our own ignorance and lack of honesty. All too often, in spite of the reassuring conventional images we have of family life, the main function of a spouse and children is to fill our own emptiness and hide our inadequacies. This is, to begin with, impossible. It is also a poor foundation on which to build a mutually nurturing family environment.

Family life at present is difficult, complex and confusing. Society quite rightly sees the family as its very foundation, yet in reality, those trying to put energy and love into it are penalized financially, both professionally and socially. In a sense the "system" is to blame, but we are part of that system and it reflects our values. Often our bosses put their interests before our family, and so do we. If we want to change the system, we need to change ourselves first. After all, we are the employer, the employee, the parent and the child.

Food and Eating

The daily activity that perhaps most requires your awareness is eating. You are literally what you eat. Think of how many times a day you drink or eat. You have been doing this, and will continue to do this, every day of your life. If the quantity or quality of what you ingest is not appropriate, even in a minor way, sooner or later you will suffer for it.

Food is a perfect example of the adage "more is less." Even a hundred years ago, Western eating habits were far different from what they are now. Food was a high priority in life because it consumed a much larger part of one's earnings. Eating was a simpler matter because there was little choice. Most food was fresh and locally (also organically) grown; what was available depended on the season. Eating habits were stable because there was little food importation and processing. Sugar was a luxury item, as were dairy and animal products. Annual sugar consumption in the West was about 4 pounds per person at the beginning of this century; now, with a "higher" standard of living, it is about 140 pounds!

In developed Western nations, food has become a priority in another sense — it represents a major health risk. While many people in the world, even within our own countries, still go hungry, we have almost too much quantity and variety; we can eat a fresh mango in the middle of a snowstorm. Unfortunately, we also have to worry about calories, cholesterol, fats, oils, sodium, colourings, preservatives, pesticides, synthetics and industrial pollutants.

As usual, we are choking on our own complexity. We have so many options in both production and consumption, we do not know where to turn. Should food be as cheap as possible or is the quality of food and the long-term care of the land more important? Are we thinking too much or not enough about what we eat? Which nutritional theory is correct? Should we subsidize farmers? Should food be used as a political weapon?

Insight Meditation starts not with theoretical answers but with immediate, practical questions. What is the purpose of eating? What is determining how and what you are eating at this very moment? What, when and why we eat is rarely determined by the body's needs, but rather by the mind's whims. "Do I have time?" "What is the quickest and cheapest food to prepare?" "What do I like eating the most?" "What coincides with my theory of nutrition?" "What will give me the most comfort?" "What is my traditional food?" "What is socially or politically correct?"

Food fills not just the stomach but also strong emotional and psychological needs. If you feel empty, unloved or threatened, you can use food, with its powerful symbolic associations, to comfort yourself. You can try to fill up the feelings of emptiness; you can use layers of flesh to keep emotions in check or to protect yourself from the outside world. Food can temporarily soothe the effects of your conflicts and suffering, but they often create other problems. Food cannot resolve your conflicts.

The only way out of this dilemma (as with any other) is not more effort and theory, but more space and mindfulness. If the main purpose of eating is to nourish the body, then listen to the body. The body has information and is less tricky than the mind. It can tell you what is healthy and what is not.

Begin your mindfulness of eating as soon as you feel hungry or start thinking about food. Is it the body needing nourishment or is the mind seeking some gratification and pacification? Is your eating merely the force of habit? If you feel yourself being swept away by compulsion, keep on looking so that you can see how the compulsion operates in both body and mind. If you find yourself fighting compulsion, then that process, too, must be observed. If you look carefully, you will see that neither submission nor willpower work in the long run, since they both remain within the realm of duality. Only choiceless, total, non-attached action — non-action — works.

The next stage in the process of mindfulness is to watch yourself as you acquire your food, either while cooking at home or eating out. What criteria do you use when selecting your food? Are they appropriate? Do you really have a choice or are you driven by compulsion? If you are cooking your own food, use it as a separate body mindfulness practice, as described in the preceding section on housework.

It is a good idea to eat slowly and mindfully. Look at yourself slowly pick up the food; smell it; taste it as you place it in your mouth; chew it slowly and well; swallow it mindfully and feel it entering your body. Generally, the slower you eat, the less you eat. Eating slowly is also better for your digestion. Watch out for restlessness while eating — tapping your fingers on the table, wanting to read, listening to the radio or watching television. Eat the food, not the "menu" or the idea about how the food is supposed to be.

The final phase in mindfulness of eating is to pay attention to the after-effects of eating. How do the mind and the body react after your meal? Is there a craving for more food? Are there any alterations in your state of mind, energy or body? Do you have more or less energy? Do you feel elated or depressed?

It is not unusual for Vipassana meditators to lose significant amounts of weight without even trying. As they begin to understand their patterns and compulsions in connection with eating, food is used less frequently to satisfy emotional needs. They also begin to see clearly how the quality of food affects their energy level, state of mind and their overall health. They accordingly seek out more healthy and appropriate ways of eating.

Others, however, change neither the quantity nor quality of what they eat and still lose weight. I regard these as examples of a phenomenon that I had noticed before — namely, that the body is a reflection of the mind, and if something deep changes in the mind, the body will reflect it. Thus, if the mind gives up its "baggage," so does the body; if the mind becomes more trusting of its environment, then the body lightens up, giving up its "armour"; if the mind becomes more balanced and alive, flowing with the currents of life, so does the body. The body becomes neither hard nor soft, heavy nor light, but just right. It is finally allowed to follow its natural instincts without interference from the mind.

Mind-Body Exercises

In our increasingly sedentary urban environment, the body needs special exercises to keep it in good working order. As with eating, however, it is usually the mind that decides for the body what is good for it. Currently, the most popular exercises train the body to tolerate increasing amounts of stress and punishment, often with the aim of shaping the body according to the mind's ideals. In essence, most of us exercise to look good in other people's eyes rather than to develop the health and balance that our particular system requires. This may not necessarily result in the current cultural ideal of a slim and taut body or one bulging with muscles.

Another aspect of this type of exercise that we should ponder is that it is a form of stress. The body accommodates itself to the demands being made on it, whether this consists of lifting weights or running long distances. In this respect, it is as good to bear in mind the three phases of Hans Selye's stress syndrome. If we continue subjecting ourselves to stress, we deplete our adaptation energy and may fall into the disintegration phase. It does not surprise me that people who train intensively look drawn, stringy and prematurely aged.

The body has considerable intelligence of its own that in some areas is superior to that of the mind. For example, when running long distances, the body can distinguish between ordinary discomfort and genuine warning signals. The mind is capable of imposing its will so tyrannically that some marathon runners have literally run themselves to death.

Some time should be set aside each day for exercises that encourage the mind and body to work in harmony. Tai Chi and yoga immediately spring to mind. They are slow enough for the mind to pay attention to each detail and gentle enough to do no violence to the body. They encourage supple and natural movement.

Both Tai Chi and yoga accumulate the intrinsic life energies, "chi" or "pranna," and circulate them throughout the body. These energies have enormous healing qualities. It would take a whole book to describe either Tai Chi Chuan or yoga. Suffice to say that they both work on the levels of mind, body and energy. Tai Chi Chuan, in addition, is a highly effective martial art that stresses continuous outward movement coexistent with a still, unmoving centre. Tai Chi Chuan is a remarkable physical manifestation of yin-yang philosophy. In practising it, we can experience what it is like to be still yet moving, to be complex yet simple, to be soft yet powerful, to retreat yet advance, to be inside and outside at the same time. To practise Tai Chi Chuan properly, you must be totally in the moment, with mind and body unified and working in powerful, intelligent harmony. Tai Chi Chuan, like Vipassana, is an ongoing journey. Each moment is different and new. There can be no stopping.

VI

A GUIDE TO
PERSONALITY

*"My life has been permeated and held together by one idea
and one goal: namely, to penetrate into the secret of personality. Everything can be explained from this central point."*
— CARL JUNG

Insight Meditation is open-ended and ongoing. You
can set up certain routines to help you apply your practice, but you can never be sure where that practice
will take you. Looking at yourself without goals or judgement is like taking the cover off a boiling cauldron —
you never know what will bubble up to the surface next.

In the two chapters that follow, I touch on several
fundamental issues that are liable to arise at some time
or other during your journey of self-discovery. They
can plague you all your life if you do not learn to
resolve the conflicts inherent in them.

Personality

Conditioning, as I have described it in several contexts,
is the accumulation of the past — memories, behavioural
patterns, experiences, beliefs, judgements, likes and dislikes, self-images, and so on — that causes us to react
in a compulsive, automatic fashion. It is very difficult to
free yourself from conditioning, because you identify
with it. It is your "I," and as such, it is self-defensive and
self-sustaining; it craves security and control.

If you practise Insight Meditation skilfully, you will begin to see your particular conditioning patterns first-hand. You will realize that your behaviour is not as random or free-willed as you first believed. You will see small and large fragments of your conditioning patterns emerging.

In time, you may discover that several of these patterns and processes are themselves organized into a consistent unity or "personality," almost like a separate person (or persons) living inside your body. There is a growing area of study and treatment that focuses on common sub-personalities and archetypes, such as the Inner Child, the Wild Man, the Goddess, the Crone. It is a fascinating and increasingly popular subject.

In my experience, we each have a general or overriding personality that is stronger and more consistent than the sub-personalities. This is not to deny the importance of the sub-personalities, which are often (but not necessarily) part of the patterns of the overall personality. Amazingly, these general personality types are not random but seem to fall into just nine basic patterns. If this is indeed true, then a knowledge of the basic personality types would obviously be an invaluable tool in piecing together the many patterns of conditioning that you may see arising during your Insight Meditation practice.

It must be pointed out that mere intellectual knowledge of the personality types is insufficient to bring about real change. You will still be deeply identified with these patterns, even if they are destructive. Freeing yourself from the compulsion of personality, or any other form of conditioning, is the domain of Vipassana or its equivalent. Knowledge is always but a tool.

The Enneagram Personality Types
The Enneagram, unlike most other personality typologies, is not based on modern psychological theories.

It is a body of knowledge from an ancient, mystic (probably Sufi) tradition that, until recently, was passed on orally by spiritual teachers. It was used to help seekers of self-knowledge understand some of their main conditioning patterns.

I first heard of the system in the late 1970s from my meditation master, Dhiravamsa, who was a friend of one of the first American teachers of the Enneagram, Claudio Naranjo. Several books on the personality types of the Enneagram have recently been published with great success because readers everywhere recognize the validity of its startling insights and because it is finding increasing correlation with modern psychology-based typologies.

Like many people, I was sceptical at first of the notion that all of humanity falls into nine convenient behavioural boxes. I did not take a serious interest in the Enneagram until I trained with Dhiravamsa on San Juan Island. At that time, my wife and I were struggling with our first (and at that time only) child, Shu-Wen. Although only two years old, she was extremely demanding and would never give in, sometimes crying for an hour or more until she got her way. Dhiravamsa, sensing our difficulties, suggested that Shu-Wen might be a #8 personality, the Boss. He explained that #8s sought power and tended not to listen, so that sometimes you had to shout to get their attention!

This was not the kind of advice we would get in a child-care manual, but it immediately made us feel better because we had been shouting at her. Once we understood her way of thinking, we could speak her (robust) language. Within weeks, there was a noticeable and positive change in the dynamics of our relationship. She started, and has continued, to become softer and gentler, which is what the Enneagram would predict of a healthy #8.

In the following pages I will outline each of the nine personality types. These patterns usually affect all our major decisions and many of the trivial ones, even down to the way we dress. There are other forms of major conditioning not covered by one's personality type, for example, parental, racial and ideological. These, however, are usually neither as deep nor as pervasive as personality.

According to the Enneagram, the complex patterns of personality revolve around a single — and false — perspective on life. This perspective, represented by one of the nine points on the circle, is so deeply in-grained that the person with that perspective usually feels it to be universal. In other words, the point on the circle (individuality) is mistaken for the whole circle (totality). We lose sight of our own limitations. We are caught in the dualistic trap described earlier: seeing our individuality but not our wholeness and our oneness.

Insight Meditation is the process of freeing your-self from all conditioning and patterns, irrespective of their source or intensity.

The Enneagram is a map of the major patterns that you are likely to encounter on your journey through life. Having a map is most helpful, but it does not replace the actual travelling, which you must undertake one mindful step at a time. Be careful not to blindly label or "box" others, or yourself; use the Enneagram as an aid to your mindfulness practice, not as a substi-tute for it. Never use the Enneagram to manipulate others, because in so doing, you harm them as well as yourself. The resentment that some people feel in being "boxed" by personality typologies is usually ego reaction. Our "I" likes to think of itself as free, unique and special. If your behaviour is easily predicted, how-ever, it means that you are predictable. You are react-ing according to a pattern; you are not exercising your free will as you think you are.

The recognition that you are indeed not free can clear the way for real change. You cannot change if you do not see the need for change. Personality is a relationship vehicle. It is no more limiting or "boxing" than your physical vehicle, your body. Both the personality and the body are tools to be used; they should not be allowed to assume the role of user.

Personality #1: The Perfectionist

The deluded perspective of the #1 personality is perfection. Most #1s immediately have a picture in their minds as to how something is to be or ought to be done. They feel that there is only one correct way and that everyone should try their utmost to attain it.

The compulsion to bring "order" to everything around them makes #1s controlling, competitive and extremely hard-working. They equate effort with self-repression, often trying to pull themselves up by their own bootstraps. They tend to put people second to principle and to regard the present human condition as a deterioration of a "golden age" that once existed. The #1 personality is that of the pioneer, the patriarch and the conservative.

Many teachers are #1s. They can maintain discipline and foster a respect for authority. They are generally moral, honest and direct, with a capacity for great detail and precision (although this is not necessarily easy for them). They are self-reliant, with their energies focused on their own families or social groupings.

On the negative side, #1s suffer from accumulated resentment and anger. They tend to be critical of themselves and of others because everything falls short of perfection. They feel frustrated but cannot express this frustration, because that is not the "correct" way to act. They tend towards "muscular armouring" — suppressing and bottling up their feelings in their bodies. Under pressure, they may explode with anger or else withdraw and sink into depression.

In meditation, #1s tend to experience physical discomfort and pain. It is difficult for them to acknowledge the "messiness" and imperfection of their own emotions, which thus remain bottled up in their bodies. They can become frustrated, feeling that they are not meditating in the "right" way or that their bodies are too pained to allow them to continue.

#1s need to learn to relax and not take things so seriously. The key to this is the realization that things and people do not have to be perfect to be worthwhile and satisfying. Perfection is only an idea that arises within them; it is not a universal commandment. Everything will be all right even without the controlling efforts of the #1.

Famous #1s include George Bernard Shaw, Martin Luther, Margaret Thatcher and Confucius, a primary source of inspiration in the Chinese culture. Another #1, the Toronto Blue Jays pitcher Dave Stieb, summed up this personality's dilemma in the title of his autobiography, *Tomorrow, I'll be Perfect*. In truth, tomorrow never comes. There is only the present.

Personality #2: The Helper, The Independent
The false perspective of the #2 personality is freedom/independence. The irony is that these types are dependent personalities, very much concerned with how people view them. They need approval and affection from others, which they usually get by being attractive and helpful. Although they may succeed in making certain people dependent on them (thus feeding their own illusions of power and independence), they are essentially dependent, garnering their feelings of self-worth from outside.

#2s are often excellent care-givers, therapists and companions. They are considerate, supportive and good listeners. They establish rapport easily on a one-on-one basis, and they go out of their way to be helpful and to meet others' needs and expectations.

They are good at blending in. They may dress and behave differently to suit various occasions and environments. Most #2s are fun to be with — enthusiastic, entertaining and alive. Many people think of them as living saints and readily confide in them.

The price of all this giving, however, is often the denial or repression of their own needs. They may become resentful, feeling that they are being taken advantage of or are not appreciated enough. To try to assert their independence, they may rebel against those on whom they most depend; they may explode in fits of anger. They tend to fall ill as a result of taking on too much or as an (often unconscious) excuse to stop taking care of others and to get some attention themselves.

#2s are proud, seeing themselves as giving help, not needing it. Even constructive criticism may be taken as an affront or an attack because their self-esteem is fragile and it originates outside themselves. They need security but shy away from true intimacy and commitment because these threaten their sense of independence.

In meditation, #2s have great difficulty with their pride and their need to feel independent. They may feel "I can do it on my own, in my own way," "I don't need help, I can help others," "Don't tell me what to do, I can manage, I know."

To free themselves from their trap, #2s first need to acknowledge their dependence and their need for approval and security. This is difficult for them because of their pride and their attachment to their self-image. If they can take this first step, they will be able to set about finding true independence within themselves. They will begin to see themselves as truly unique and special, and will not need anyone else to tell them they are. They will be capable of giving without wanting anything in return.

Examples of the #2 personality are Mother Teresa, Cher, Marilyn Monroe and Leo Buscaglia.

Personality #3: The Performer, The Success

The false perspective of the #3 personality is efficiency and success. Whereas #2s seek approval from others through being helpful and attractive, the #3 personality seeks it through peer group recognition for his or her hard work, efficiency and success.

The #3 personality is perhaps the most admired in North American culture. It is that of the businessperson, the salesperson, the agent, the manager, the facilitator, the liberal intellectual, the yuppie, the creator of consumer "packages" and the media manipulator. #3s like non-stop activity. They are aggressive, persuasive, presentable and good performers in the sense of both acting out a role (even a spiritual one) and of seeing something through to its seemingly "successful" conclusion.

The trap for this personality, like that for the #2, is that no matter how well they do, they still depend on others for their self-esteem. They must keep trying to win it over and over. Success for the #3 is as much quantitative as qualitative, so they are constantly on the lookout for new ventures. The #3s are the Type A personality often described in popular stress jargon. When #3s disintegrate, they tend to become numb, lacking energy and motivation, as in the Epstein-Barr syndrome or "yuppie flu."

The key to the success of #3s, their greatest asset, is also their greatest liability. Because of their capacity to completely identify with their roles, their jobs and their functions, they are generally very successful. The price they pay is the loss of their own souls. They lose touch with the deeper part of themselves, often denying completely the possibility of anything other than what is superficially apparent. They thus tend towards materialism.

Just as the role in life takes precedence over the "inner" self of the #3, so their work generally takes precedence over their family life. #3s tend to spend a lot of time away from home.

Insight Meditation rarely attracts #3s. Being still is difficult for them, and the prospect of delving into the dark, mysterious recesses of themselves with no immediate pay-back is not at all appealing. They need constant proof of "success." If they are attracted to spiritual matters, it is usually in a more structured and packaged form.

A few years ago, a man who turned out to be a #3 personality asked me to give him private lessons in Insight Meditation. He said that the rest of his life was in good shape and now was the time to tackle the spiritual. After just ten minutes of sitting meditation, he shouted loudly. At the end of the session, he explained that it had been the most horrible experience of his life. When I enquired what it was in particular that bothered him, he replied, "Sitting quietly. I have never done that before." He did not return for the second session because he felt he was a "failure." He would look for something more "suitable."

#3s need to slow down and look beyond the image and beyond the satisfaction of their own success. Relationship with others and with life itself needs to be built on deeper foundations than plaudits and accolades. Yet this is difficult for #3s because society rewards them so highly for the roles they play. Those #3s who do manage to start balancing themselves tend to broaden their outlook, paying more attention to their families and to society in general. They start to look inward, beyond the compelling image they have cultivated.

Famous #3s include Laurence Olivier, Walt Disney, Werner Erhard (the founder of EST) and Ron Hubbard.

Personality #4: The Tragic-Romantic, The Artist
The deluded perspective of the #4 personality is rationalization. They constantly attempt to make some sense of their lives by replaying it over and over in their heads, wondering where they went wrong and how they can

get it right in the future. They see themselves as having been singled out by life for a tragic existence, filled with recurring loss and abandonment.

Their preoccupation with this sense of tragedy often leads them to depression and melancholy. The latter is a bitter-sweet experience, in which they can indulge themselves, often expressing it artistically or dramatically. Although melancholy is the bane of their lives, they are strongly attached to it because it makes them feel special and often creative.

#4s are generally artistic and creative with a taste for the refined and the dramatic. They see themselves as somehow apart from the mainstream. They are generally striking and attractive, but in an aloof manner; they are often the arbiters of "good taste," but in a slightly unconventional way.

Many writers, painters, high-fashion models and members of the creative community are #4s. They set the standards, often equating creativity with suffering. Japan and England exhibit strong #4 personality national traits — a strong dramatic and literary tradition, an aristocracy that has known better days, preoccupation with refinement and good taste, a sense of being misunderstood or underappreciated. These countries are also both islands — apart from the mainland, cut off.

The trap for the #4 personality is authenticity. While they are seeking the "real" meaning of life in their heads, life itself flows past them. They look down at "ordinary" people, yet at the same time envy them; they want but do not take.

It is difficult for #4s to let go of their melancholy and depression. These black moods make them feel different and are often the inspiration for their creative endeavours. #4s are so trapped in their heads that they often lose touch with their bodies and may become physically and mentally disoriented. This confusion often derives from the many mental scenarios that #4s write for the past as well as for the future. Under pressure, #4s may give up trying to help themselves, desperately hoping for a saviour to come along. They may occasionally become suicidal.

In meditation, #4s are usually afflicted by non-stop thinking. Some have never had the experience of not thinking and therefore are out of touch with emotions and the body. They do not *feel* emotions and physical sensations but filter them through thought. They often experience confusion and indecision, not knowing where to turn.

There is no way out for the #4s if they hold on to their constant introspection. The real is not in their head but in the moment, in the very ordinariness of life that they shun. It is a good idea for them to start doing rather than thinking. Success through their own actions in the "real world" can be the best tonic for them. Exercise and activity are also generally beneficial for #4s, although these may seem difficult at first.

Famous #4s include Alan Watts, Joni Mitchell, John Keats, Ingmar Bergman, Meryl Streep and Percy Bysshe Shelley.

Personality #5: The Observer

The false perspective of the #5 personality is observation. #5s feel that by observing life they can determine its mechanisms and thereby control it and keep it at bay. Their observations are generally wide-ranging and often accurate, but the stance of the observer creates a distance from others and from life in general. Knowledge about life is not life.

#5 personalities can be excellent decision-makers and intellectuals. Their ability to detach themselves allows them to see people and situations with clarity and balance. The search for omniscience makes #5s collectors of bits and pieces of knowledge, which they store in cuttings, files, libraries and computers. They tend to know something about almost every subject.

Although omniscience is an admirable and valid goal, it is not life. It is *about* life. #5s use knowledge, self-denial and withdrawal as protection against involvement. They do not trust life to provide for them, so they feel they must do it themselves. They barricade themselves inside their ivory towers. The better they are at protecting themselves, the more isolated they become, and the more difficult they find it to ask for help or even to make contact with others.

If the #5's fortress is breached or their knowledge challenged, they tend to feel swamped and invaded. They suffer "psychic panic," which is a sort of claustrophobia. Most #5s need a lot of private space and time in their lives. They tend to see socializing and small talk as a waste of valuable time, during which they could be stockpiling intellectual or other goods. #5s generally dislike any form of commitment to or coercion by others.

#5s generally like Vipassana because it is based on observing. Their trap is that they may spend too much time in solitary observation and not enough getting involved in life and with people.

#5s need to give up their fortifications and set forth to meet life, not shrink from it. They need to put their elaborate strategies to the test in the heat of life's battles; they need to exercise their power instead of theorizing about it; they need to start trusting their gut feelings.

Famous #5s include Albert Einstein, Franz Kafka, Albert Camus, Glenn Gould, J. Paul Getty and Howard Hughes.

Personality #6: The Adventurer, The Loyalist
The false perspective of the #6 personality is adventure. Because they are plagued by anxiety and self-doubt, they seek to prove themselves in one situation after another or to find that one person, group or system that they hope will forever put their fears and indecision to rest.

#6s are good at working against the odds. They are generally anti-authoritarian and, once they have given their loyalty to a cause or to a person, steadfast. They can be hard-working, self-sacrificing and sometimes capable of astonishing mind-over-matter feats. These qualities make them loyal and valuable friends and team members. Many soldiers, police officers, mountaineers and marathon runners are #6s.

The #6 personality can exhibit patterns of behaviour that seem in total contradiction to each other. There are actually two types of #6s, the Phobic and the Counter-phobic. The Phobic is furtive, anxious and full of self-doubt, like Woody Allen. A Counter-phobic, like Oliver North, may seem confident, challenging or even abrasive, camouflaging fear with antagonistic behaviour and compulsive bravery. #6s may alternate bouts of loyalty and stability with bouts of constant seeking and experimentation.

In spite of their appearance, #6s are basically fearful, especially of authority figures. They are given to projection and even paranoia; they are constantly on the lookout for possible threats. They try to combat their fears with compulsive bravery and to conceal their indecision and anxiety by adopting a stable structure, whether in the form of a person, a belief or a group. Once they have adopted a structure, they will fight to protect it because, in effect, they are protecting themselves. The army is a perfect structure for many #6s because it not only gives them something plausible to believe in and to fight for but it also gives them the opportunity to demonstrate their courage and loyalty.

The greatest challenge that #6s experience in Insight Meditation is consistency. Even if they find it eminently reasonable, there is always the temptation to move on and try to find something better. I pointed out to a #6 once that even if there was a perfect system or method, the #6 would not stay with it because there would always be the possibility of something better. She shamefacedly agreed with me. She left our group soon afterwards.

The #6 personality cannot overcome fear through compulsive bravery, but only through real courage. Real courage comes after first accepting and understanding the process of fear. If fear is denied, then there can be no way of working with it. The emphasis for the #6 personality must be on harmony and reconciliation, not on fighting.

Famous #6s include Richard Nixon, Sigmund Freud, Napoleon, Hitler and the Cowardly Lion in *The Wizard of Oz*.

Personality #7: The Idealist

The #7 personality's false perspective on life is the notion of the ideal. #7s mask their underlying fears with plans and hopes for good times, individually and collectively. They are compulsive optimists, with their heads in the clouds. They tend to ignore the dark side of reality and often have difficulty implementing their plans.

#7s are attractive. They tend to be eloquent, entertaining speakers, with perpetual grins and beautiful visions of the future. They like participating in groups, both to reinforce their own ideals and to promote togetherness and good times. Balanced #7s use their enthusiasm and their organizational and communication skills to good effect within large organizations.

Internationalist political parties, charities, ecological groups, growth centres, cooperatives and other idealistic ventures usually contain a high percentage of #7 personality types. The hippie counter-culture of the 1960s was a good example of the #7 personality in action, as are many present-day new age spiritual groups and organizations that emphasize togetherness, feeling good and movement towards the "light."

Unfortunately, insisting that the world is rose-coloured does not make it so. Problems do not go away by themselves. Underlying fears cannot be totally or permanently glossed over by positive thinking. Our Shadow or dark side will not be denied or ignored. #7s tend to confuse talking about something with the experience of the thing itself. In the realm of spirituality, they tend to see themselves as very advanced or even enlightened. They have difficulty in implementing plans and in fulfilling commitments, which they avoid as much as possible.

When the gap between reality and their ideals becomes too large to ignore, they may become resentful and aggressive, trying to bend reality to fit their ideals. Alternatively, they may just walk away from it all. The latter course may be a physical departure or an internal escape through drugs or through narcissistic self-preoccupation.

In the practice of Insight Meditation, #7s have a lot of difficulty with the physical or emotional pain that may be revealed. Unless this is dealt with, it will remain trapped by unfounded optimism, gathering force and darkness.

Instead of being so intent on having a good time and fashioning beautiful dreams, #7s would benefit by allowing themselves to stay in the present. By taking a long, unbiased look at themselves and their environment, a more balanced view of life would emerge. They would not then be so afraid of confronting pain and discomfort. Thus strengthened and balanced, they would be much more successful in implementing their inspirational visions.

Famous #7s include Ram Dass, Joan Rivers, Peter Pan and James Joyce.

Personality #8: The Boss, The Justice-Maker
The false perspective of the #8 personality is justice. #8s see the world as a hostile environment where justice must be enforced through strength. They seek power

so that they can stand up for themselves and for those under their protection to ensure that justice is done.

Many leaders and bosses are #8s. They not only gravitate towards positions of power but are often physically strong and imposing. They tend to be combative, assertive and forceful, generally unselfconscious about displaying anger. They respect those who have the courage to stand up to them. Balanced #8s make excellent leaders and campaigners for those who have been wronged.

Although #8s are good at fighting external enemies, they are not so skilled at combating the internal ones. They tend to avoid or suppress anything within themselves that they associate with weakness — tenderness, sensitivity, compassion, yielding. In so doing, they choke off their capacity to love and be loved; they isolate themselves. #8s try to fill this self-created void with sensual excess — sex, alcohol, drugs or food.

#8s also avoid introspection because it might undermine their simplistic notions of right and wrong. #8s like a clearly defined target on which to focus. They want to know who are the "good guys" and who are the "bad guys." In their minds, they are, of course, the good guys.

Unfortunately, no matter how powerful they are, self-esteem is still seen by most #8s as something outside themselves. They are in the same dilemma as the #2 personality. While the #2 personality tries to win that self-esteem from others through being helpful and charming, the #8 seizes it forcefully.

In Vipassana, #8s have difficulty acknowledging weakness. They are so accustomed to being in control and to giving orders that they cannot be open to the new and the unexpected. No one, however, is all-powerful. We all have weaknesses, and that is not necessarily bad. In Tai Chi Chuan, the soft ultimately overcomes the hard.

#8s need to see the value of softness and sensitivity. They have to learn to give as well as to take, to truly listen as well as to command. Only in this way will they be able to experience a loving two-way relationship and to realize a deeper meaning of the word "justice."

Famous #8s include Gurdjieff, Fritz Perls (the creator of Gestalt therapy), Nietzsche, Pablo Picasso, Ernest Hemingway and Katharine Hepburn.

Personality #9: The Peace-Maker

The deluded perspective of the #9 personality is non-conformity. This might seem strange at first, since most #9s appear highly conventional. They are, however, nonconformists in the sense that they are always seeking ways of achieving peace and harmony and of becoming more decisive. Although being "settled" is one of their main goals in life, they can allow themselves to be led into new and different (nonconforming) experiences because they are not truly satisfied with their lives.

#9 personality types also have an aptitude for and attraction to routine, detailed, impersonal work. They tend to avoid any stressful decision-making, unsettling self-promotion or unpredictable interactions with others. Many accountants, bureaucrats and dentists are #9s.

The price #9s pay for being able to see others' points of view so clearly is that they neglect their own. They have little feeling of self-worth and therefore have difficulty asserting themselves and taking the initiative. They are generally not good self-starters. They tend to wait for others to draw them into activity, creative or otherwise. If this does not happen, they may sedate themselves in trivia or mindless routine, perhaps becoming "couch potatoes." Under pressure, they may become more anxious and indecisive, looking for some belief or structure to grasp, similar to the unhealthy aspect of the #6 personality.

#9s tend to fall asleep a lot during their sitting meditation practice. Their minds go to sleep to avoid seeing anything upsetting or disturbing.

#9s need to realize that true peace is not indolence or the lack of external turbulence. It is something that arises inside themselves often only after turbulence and conflict are faced and understood. They would benefit by stirring themselves, setting goals and achieving them. It is healthy for them to open their hearts to the unpredictability of love and relationships.

Well-known #9s include Buckminster Fuller, Alfred Hitchcock, Dwight Eisenhower and Ringo Starr.

The above are, of course, mere thumb-nail sketches of the nine personality types. Yet if you have an understanding of the basic dynamics of each personality type, you can understand their infinite variations and how they relate to other forms of conditioning. The overwhelming majority of people have only one personality in their lifetime. It exerts a strong influence most of the time, even if other forms of conditioning seem to be manifesting themselves on the surface.

A woman who attended one of my Enneagram personality workshops was surprised to discover that she had spent most of her life (she was in her early forties) acting like a #2 personality when she was actually a #3. She had idolized her mother, a #2, and had tried to be giving and caring, even becoming a nurse. It was only in the year before attending the workshop that her #3 personality had finally broken through to the surface. She had given up nursing to start her own business. Although she was greatly relieved to have found her "true" self, I pointed out that unfortunately this "true" self was itself just another mask — only a point on the circle, not the circle itself.

Religion, philosophy, culture and specialized environments (such as type of job) can likewise act as a personality overlay, identifiable in accordance with the Enneagram. This should not be surprising since all great philosophers and teachers necessarily express their ideas or insights through the vehicle of their personality. The Chinese culture, for example, is heavily influenced by Confucius, who was a #1 personality type. Many Chinese display strong #1 personality traits, like hard work, honesty, competitiveness, putting principle before the individual, a reverence for tradition and an emphasis on family life. This does not mean that all Chinese are #1 personality types, but that Chinese are very influenced by their "Chineseness."

Many sub-groups in society display a collective personality simply because people of the same type are drawn to the same activities and environments. Thus the teaching profession is heavily influenced by #1-type attitudes and thinking, nursing and social work by #2s, business and the media by #3s, the artistic community by #4s, psychoanalytic therapy and academia by #5s, the army and the police force by #6s, "green" politics and new age spirituality by #7s, the legal profession by #8s, and dentistry and accountancy by #9s. While it is comforting to be among like-minded people, there is the danger that shared conditioning will be mistaken for universal truth. This is especially pernicious in spiritual circles where the avowed goal is universal truth.

Although intellectual knowledge of the Enneagram personality patterns can be a powerful tool, it is nevertheless limited. The intellect, as we have seen, can help you distinguish constituent parts, but it is not very good at integrating those parts. It can help you understand your patterns of behaviour, but it cannot free you from those patterns because of its own identification with them.

Freeing ourselves from conditioning, personality or otherwise, is the work of Insight Meditation or some equivalent. The Enneagram can help in this process because if you recognize your action as part of a pattern, then you know conditioning must be at work. The more conditioned, predictable and rigid you are, the less immediate and alive will be your response to life.

VII

RELATIONSHIPS

"Existence is relationship; to be is to be related. Relationship is society. The structure of our present society, being based on mutual use, brings about violence, destruction and misery."
— *J.D. KRISHNAMURTI*

"When unobstructed relationship occurs between individuals, both people have released subject/object consciousness. This is the most remarkable of all relationships. One can call it archetypal because in that moment each person sees the other as themselves and simultaneously whole."
— *RICHARD MOSS, M.D.*

No one is an island. The atomic physicists tell us so, and with near-instantaneous global communication, it is becoming increasingly difficult to sustain the illusion of even national boundaries.

In that sense, it can be said that you are always in relationship — with your loved ones, your work associates, your friends and acquaintances, your government, your country and your planet. Your every action affects others (even if you choose to do nothing), and their actions affect you. The closer the relationship, the stronger is the effect.

If you want to improve your relationships (that is, bring about positive change), the most effective action you can take is to change yourself. You can never really change another person, although you may at times influence their behaviour through coercion or manipulation. The Buddha pointed out that even Buddhas (perfectly enlightened beings) can only show the way. The essential work of transformation must be done by the individual alone. Both Jesus and the Buddha said very little about how to regulate society. Instead, they directed their teachings at the source of humanity's transformation, the individual.

In our present state of consciousness, our actions predominantly originate from the mental ego or "I." Since the primary function of the ego is to sustain and enlarge itself, it follows that all other considerations are secondary. In the last resort, "my" interests always seem more pressing and justifiable than "yours." We are open-minded as long as the other person does not threaten our core beliefs; we are charitable as long as we have a surplus (say of wealth or power) for ourselves and the recipient of our charity is appropriately grateful; we are loving as long as our love object does what we want; we are reasonable as long as the other person accepts our reasoning. If "my" interests ultimately take precedence over yours, then our relationship must be based on usage. Mutual usage or usage sanctioned by society, religion, custom, tradition, whatever, does not alter the basic fact of usage.

We do not even bother to hide the exploitative nature of our relationship with our environment. We regard everything on the face of the planet as ours for the taking, even if that entails unwarranted waste, destruction and killing. The major restraint on our abuse of the planet is not conscience but the greed and self-interest of competing humans.

If we look beyond our high-sounding rationalizations, we cannot fail to see this same attitude of exploitation permeating our relationships with our fellow human beings. Slavery is still with us; war is still with us; trade and business is unabashedly based on exploitation. In fact, we routinely present ourselves as commodities not only in the workplace but in relationships. The element of usage is also present, though in a subtler way, in many seemingly healthy relationships such as husband and wife, teacher and student, guru and disciple.

If we acknowledge that most of our actions are essentially "me first," then what we see around us should not be surprising. We cannot truly love if we need something in return; we cannot lead others to clarity if we ourselves are confused and in conflict; we cannot build a just and compassionate society if our own self-interests are paramount; we cannot truly give if we want to receive. Some Third World countries no longer accept Western "aid" because they find the attached strings too costly in the long run.

To really change your life and the essential dynamics of your relationships, you must shift the source of your actions from the "I" to that which is deeper and more universal. This shift gives rise to what we have discussed as non-action — action that is whole, harmonious and undistorted by individual ego. This shift takes much courage and perseverance and is a task that each individual must perform for himself or herself, since it requires self-knowledge. Carl Jung wrote, "The individual who wishes to have an answer to the problem of evil, has need, first and foremost of self-knowledge, that is, the utmost possible knowledge of his wholeness. He must know relentlessly how much good he can do and what crimes he is capable of . . . Both are elements within his nature, and both are bound to come to light in him, should he wish — as he ought to — to live without self-deception or self-delusion."

There can be no half-measures in the process of transformation. A little less "me first," unfortunately, is not sufficient to do the trick; a little self-deception is still self-deception. There must be a complete shift in the source of our activity from the ego or "I." Moreover, we must embark on that process immediately. Putting it off or setting conditions for changing is not transformation but additional ego-defensive manoeuvring.

Although self-preservation is a natural law, our interpretation of "self" is extremely limited. Our true self includes that which we do not regard as self. It also includes the "other," not only our partner, our children and our friends but our enemies and even non-human species; it includes our planet. The more limited our sense of self, the more fearful, suffocated and vulnerable we are. The larger our sense of self, the more expansive, accommodating, trusting and resilient we are. This process must not be confused with the ego's attempt to enlarge itself through power or identification.

Unfortunately, we cannot move from "me first" action to non-action by a simple effort of will. That too would be ego-derived and would serve only to complicate matters. We must learn to let go of our attachments (which might include people, things, beliefs, desires) when necessary. We must keep on coming back to the present and acknowledging the distortions and conflicts taking place in our lives. By letting go of distortions, conflicts and fragmentations, one by one, we automatically move away from the confinements of the "I." We free ourselves to move towards clarity, wholeness and unobstructed relationship.

Men and Women

The current battle between the sexes is more serious than is generally acknowledged. It is more like a war. Women, having been subservient to men for so long, understandably will not be denied power. Power, however, is rarely surrendered voluntarily.

As in any war, there is not only great turmoil and confusion but bitterness, hatred and excess. In any battle, there is a tendency to stick with your own kind in order to battle the "enemy." Both men and women are suffering because of this tendency.

This is sad, because in reality there is no enemy. Fighting, at any level or for any cause, may bring a redistribution of power, but it does not resolve conflict. In this case, it resolves neither the tension between men and women nor the other problems that we all face as human beings. We remain caught in duality — making effort and progress, but never getting there.

How is Vipassana relevant to this complex conflict? It can bring clarity and harmony in each moment. It allows you to cut through the righteous rhetoric of both the traditionalists and the current arbiters of politically correct gender-think. More important than man or woman, homosexual or heterosexual, black or white, is human. If you are able to treat the other person as an equal human being, most problems disappear.

In thinking about female-male, I find it helpful to go back to the yin-yang diagram. The difference between the opposites is plainly and non-judgementally acknowledged — one is black and one is white. One is not preferable to the other. Women are fundamentally different from men. They do not need to be "mannish" to exercise power just because, in the past, power was mostly exercised by men. They do not need suits, padded shoulders or hard-muscled bodies; they do not need to deny their natural physiology; they certainly do not need workaholism and death by cigarette.

The yin-yang diagram also reveals that yin contains a measure of yang, and vice versa. Women can be soft and yielding, but it is healthy for them to be assertive when necessary; they have that inherent power. Many men tend to be more rigid and aggressive, but need softness for balance. Learning how to be vulnerable and how to nurture is crucial.

Some would consider my statements outrageous stereotyping. If these people were familiar with the theory and practice of Tai Chi, they would realize that soft and yielding is often far superior to hard and aggressive. At present, men and women alike tend to scorn or underestimate the power to yield and to accept. That is why we are all knocking heads.

There is a time and place for everything. Nothing and no one is inherently good or bad, right or wrong. Yin and yang are always seeking to be in balance with each other and will achieve it if left to flow naturally. Yin and yang are different, yet always the same.

Partners

My dictionary defines *partner* as "one who is associated with another or others in the enjoyment or possession of anything; a partaker, sharer." This is a very wide definition, and today we are seeing an ever-widening diversity in relationships — from traditional marriages to relationships in which all the specific terms, stipulations and penalty clauses are set forth in legal documents, very much as in commercial agreements. Marriage has almost always been a form of contract. The terms of traditional marriages were determined mostly by religious and social considerations. The terms of modern marriages or relationships are determined increasingly by the partners themselves, either formally, in a contract, or subconsciously through the interaction of their personalities.

Whatever the specific terms, however, most long-term relationships are based on expectation and trade-off. You give up something — mostly independence — to get something else in return — mostly that illusive "security" in its many forms. If you do not get what you bargained for, you feel cheated. You become angry or depressed. Eventually the relationship dies, whether you actually walk away or not.

Most relationships start off well enough. Everything is new and exciting. There may be infatuation, passion and the sheer novelty of learning to share your life with another. There is also a life-long succession of projects to keep you busy: saving up for a house (then ever bigger and better houses), climbing social and career ladders, having children and planning for retirement.

Initially, because most marriages are based on complementarity, it may seem the ideal solution to life's problems. If you find certain challenges difficult, if you lack certain qualities or sense certain voids in your life, why not marry someone who will live out those deficient parts for you? It is no coincidence that often one partner is introverted and the other outgoing, one giving and the other taking, one rigid and the other yielding, one the parent figure and the other the child. Much of the attraction between partners is, consciously or subconsciously, based on a search for completeness and wholeness.

Sooner or later, couples encounter the same problems and limitations as individuals. There is the gap between what is and what you want or expect; there is the boredom and restlessness that arises from repetition. No matter how hard you try, there is a feeling of incompleteness and emptiness; you always need more to fill you up.

Life is continually changing, whereas we are bound to the past by our internal conditioning factors. In a relationship, each partner is weighed down by not one but two sets of patterns and experiences. Moreover, familiarity tends to breed contempt, or at least complacency. It is easy to feel you know the other person and to find a reason to blame them for whatever seems to be going wrong in your life. This often leads to the feeling that you have been misled or taken advantage of.

If you see yourself as a commodity in the relationship business, then the logical solution to any problem is to get a lawyer to secure your best financial and other interests. Trade in the old model for a new one and hope you get a good bargain. In truth, all parties to such transactions devalue their own humanity.

On the other hand, sticking with a relationship simply because you happen to find yourself in one is not a solution either. If the relationship does not enrich the lives of either of the partners and there seems little willingness by the partners to change, it is rarely wise to stay in it. Such deep conflict is debilitating and often generates great bitterness. The welfare of the children is not necessarily served by preserving such a relationship. It is perhaps better for the children to learn how to adapt to the realities of change rather than how to live a lie.

Being reasonably whole as a couple, in the sense of each partner complementing the other, does not make each partner whole as an individual. If you are not whole as an individual, then you are almost certainly using your partner to try to fill your personal voids — in terms of a lack of security, esteem, lost childhood, or lost parent. If your expectations, reasonable or unreasonable, are not met, you will feel disappointed and perhaps bitter. Consciously or subconsciously, you will try to find ways (subtle, direct, socially acceptable or otherwise) of getting even. This is inevitable if the basis of the relationship is one of usage.

Mutual dependence and usage, together with finely balanced complementarity, sometimes make for a long-lasting relationship. Even this, however, is not the ideal that people think it is. In the first place, such a balancing act is rare. Second, even if it can be accomplished, there is, as usual, a price to be paid. In order to cement the pact, the partners must in effect agree to lock themselves into an unchanging set of behavioural patterns. This is a denial of change, growth and aliveness; routine becomes important for its own sake. The partners remain extremely dependent on one another, so that if one leaves or dies, the other is devastated.

In any relationship, we must ask ourselves what is of paramount importance: the interests of the couple or of the individuals making up the couple? Those interests may not necessarily coincide. An individual cannot become whole if he or she depends on another. This does not mean that individuals should not enter into partnership, but that the possibility of partnership without usage and dependence should be explored.

There is nothing in life, including relationships, that anyone can guarantee. You may manipulate, control or give in to another, but you can never really change them. Real change can be accomplished only by the individual.

The best that you can do for any relationship is to love your partner unconditionally. If you are honest with yourself, you will see that this is extremely rare. That is why, in this book, very little is said about love. Most of us do not know true, unconditional love. You cannot move from conditional love to unconditional love through an act of will. What you can do is begin releasing yourself from those conditions that keep you acting from the space of "me first."

In the absence of unconditional love, the best you can do is try to keep your end of the relationship unobstructed and undistorted by the demands of your "I." For example, if you feel jealous but know that this feeling is unreasonable, admit it both to yourself and to your partner. Watch the feeling as it rises and falls away, much as you would during your "household Zen" meditation practice. If you can free yourself from the snare of jealousy, not only would your partnership benefit but so too would all your other relationships.

If your partner does the same, then the relationship will flow harmoniously — easily, cleanly and ever-fresh. There will be space for both partners to change and grow; there will be a willingness and an ability to resolve conflict and to adapt to new situations; each moment will be new, instead of being just a reprise of the past. There will be greater opportunity for true love to flourish because the partners will be sensitive to each other as they are in the present; they will be together because they want to be, rather than because they need to be.

The qualities required for a harmonious relationship, therefore, are exactly the same as those needed for personal growth, transformation and harmony within: clarity, lovingness, compassion and the ability to let go of attachments and let things be. For true wholeness in a relationship, each partner must be whole. If you perceive the need for change in your relationships, then start with yourself. It should at least clarify which part of the problem is yours and which is your partner's.

If one partner attempts or achieves transformation before the other, it may cause some imbalance and turbulence in the relationship. This is not necessarily a bad thing, but might provide an incentive for the other partner to seek real change too, thereby raising the relationship to a higher, less manipulative level. Unfortunately, some partners do not understand the nature or innate power of the transformation process. They may feel threatened by it and try to sabotage it, or they may leave the relationship altogether. In a sense, they are trying to run away from their own need to change, an escape that is ultimately futile. Growth and transformation are human destiny, whether they come sooner or later . . . after many more lessons in suffering.

Parents and Children

The basic qualities of clarity and compassion necessary for a nurturing relationship between partners, are also needed between parents and children. Indeed, that need is far greater because of the vulnerability of children and the intense emotions they can provoke in us. Children are often the object of extreme identification and projection, positive and negative, by parents trying to fill their own voids.

In the following discussion, it must be remembered that although we may be adults and parents, we were also once children. In fact, the child in us may still be exerting a significant influence over our lives, whether we realize it or not. In reflecting about your relationship with your children, think also about your relationship with your own parents; think about yourself.

Parents (or persons fulfilling that role) have an extremely powerful and long-lasting effect on babies and young children. Since babies are completely immobile, dependent and impressionable, the adults are the world to them. The adults' behaviour will determine whether the world is regarded as safe, trustworthy and nurturing or filled with unpredictability, neglect, suspicion, violence and horror. Do not believe for a moment that even newborn babies cannot remember. They can. All too often, however, their memory is blocked by unbearable pain and fear, their monsters trapped in their haunted unconscious.

Our perception of sexual role models and of relationship dynamics almost invariably comes from our parents. From them, we learn how men and women behave, how they interact and, very likely, how they manipulate each other. Although we will encounter other role models as we grow up, the early ones remain extremely influential.

It is difficult to escape the behavioural imprint of our parents, especially in the realm of relationships. Some children are almost undistorted reflections of their parents. Others hate what their parents did to them and attempt to do just the opposite, thereby becoming mere negative reflections of their parents. Others reflect their parents in a more complicated fashion, with male/female role reversals and with specific positive or negative reflections. Thus, a woman may hate her father (and perhaps men in general) for dominating her mother, yet in her own relationships may play a domineering role, despite seemingly submissive feminine mannerisms.

Parents are in a difficult position. Most carry the burden of their own unresolved and unacknowledged childhood pains and conflicts yet, whether they like it or not, they are the role models for their children.

Unfortunately, trying to be the good parent that you did not have is not enough. Unless you can truly free yourself from your own childhood past (which as we have seen is not easy), you will be passing on your own neurotic patterns. If you are able to look at families over several generations, you will most likely see the same problems cropping up time and again, either in their positive or negative aspects. It seems almost like a curse or something that is passed on in the genes. It is in fact passed on, because no one has broken the patterns or is even aware that patterns exist.

Parents' words and good intentions are not enough, because children rely mostly on feelings rather than intellect. If a parent's true feelings are at odds with what he or she says or does (whether or not the parent is aware of the disparity), then the child is learning not so much what the parent is consciously saying or doing but about fragmentation, deception, inconsistency and manipulation. Even though a parent sets aside "quality" time for a child, the interaction may not be as beneficial as the parent expects if that time is not freely and lovingly given.

It is important that a parent respect a child as another human being. Children are under the protection and guidance of their parents until they can take care of themselves. They are not the property of their parents. They should not be used as extensions of their parents, vehicles for the fulfilment of their needs or scapegoats for their own frustrations. Unfortunately, this type of usage is not only common, but extreme, as the many physical and sexual abuse court cases attest.

Even the accepted attitude of "wanting the best" for your children needs closer examination. Sacrificing for the welfare of your children is commendable, especially in these self-centred times. All too often, however, your sacrifice is really for yourself. It is common to hear "My child will have the best/be the smartest/the most successful/the most beautiful." We do not hear the unspoken reasons, "because he or she is a reflection of me/because he or she can achieve what I could not/because he or she is my legacy, my way of trying to cheat death."

Becoming a parent does not magically confer upon you love, understanding and wisdom. If parents cannot free themselves from their patterns (in other words, if they are incapable of real change), they will perpetuate the cycle of manipulation and abuse from generation to generation. They will pass on their own conditioning, whether this relates to their personality, their own parents, their race or their nationality.

It is difficult to truly free yourself from your childhood conditioning. Most of us still hold a vulnerable inner child (sub-personality) within ourselves. We are afraid to let it out because we are supposed to be adults and because that child frequently is in pain or terror. We generally do not want that pain to come to our consciousness, so the child remains trapped. It often disrupts our lives as a way to get the conscious attention it needs in order to be freed.

If you are still a child yourself, you can neither properly care for your children nor establish a truly adult relationship with your own parents, or with your partner. Many people in their twilight years still act out behavioural patterns established in early childhood. Clearly most of these patterns are irrelevant. Unfortunately, even the death of your parents does not free you from the influence of these patterns. Freedom can come only when those patterns are allowed to emerge into consciousness and are released through deep insight and awareness.

Quite apart from the problem of projecting our patterns onto our children, we also face the challenge of determining and meeting their special needs. Child-care manuals give you only part of the story. They will tell you the broad stages of child development, but they cannot tell you about an individual child. That is something that only the parent can determine, through direct insight undistorted by ego-interference.

Insight Meditation has greatly helped my parenting, while being a parent has in turn deepened my meditation practice. Many times I have gone against the conventional wisdom of the day and often I have been vindicated by "new" child-rearing theories and research. No theory, however, can substitute for the ability to relate to a child (or any person for that matter) as he or she really is at that moment.

Parenting is difficult if you are genuinely interested in the welfare of your children. It is a twenty-four-hour-a-day job during which you may be pushed beyond your limits many times. There is compensation, however, because it is good for your spiritual development; it forces you to come to terms with your shortcomings and to occasionally do something for someone other than yourself. You may also be lucky enough to receive pure, innocent and unconditional love.

The best we can do for our children is give them coping tools. Material possessions, belief systems and social, intellectual and physical skills are not enough. They need to learn to adapt, to meet the specific challenges of a rapidly changing environment. We cannot save them from pain, for that is our present destiny. We can, though, through our own example, show them how they can learn from suffering and eventually release themselves from it.

Relationships with Authority and the Collective

The relationship between an individual and the collective does not need to involve authority, but in our society it usually does. Many teachers, police officers, hospital staff, bureaucrats, politicians and employers invoke their authority on the grounds that they represent a greater, collective body.

The relationship with an authority figure is one of inequality. My dictionary defines *authority* as the "power or right to enforce obedience." Thus, parents have authority, but so, too, do older siblings and playground bullies.

Authority and inequality are not in themselves a problem. They are a common occurrence in nature. The problem is that when we have power, we abuse it so predictably we think that abuse is natural too — "Power tends to corrupt and absolute power corrupts absolutely." This is yet another example of "me first" relationships based on usage and exploitation. Such relationships are indeed the rule, but they need not be. It is up to us to change that.

In a relationship with authority, it is not always the more powerful party that is the culprit. Some personalities like to be led, even though it is not necessarily healthy for them. Such people may actually contribute to their own domination. Others will react and instigate a fight with an authority figure even if that person has exhibited exemplary conduct.

We can examine these mechanisms in the relationship between employer and employee, which is perhaps the most common in our adult life. As with marriage partners, this relationship of mutual usage works as long as both parties are satisfied with the contract. Since, however, there tend to be many more parties to the agreement than in a marriage and since the element of usage is much more apparent, the underlying conflicts surface more quickly and with greater animosity.

The fact that a person (whether a parent or boss) directs and gives instructions to others does not make him or her a superior person. In business, however, both bosses and employees consciously or subconsciously subscribe to this belief. This occurs through the processes of fragmentation and identification discussed earlier. The roles or functions involved, which are only intellectual concepts, are mistaken for solid reality.

Once both parties make the identification with the superior-inferior roles, an adversarial position develops. Both parties, being driven by ego, will usually try to maintain or expand their domains. Bosses will try to control, enhance prestige and make more profits. Ambitious employees will attempt to aggressively "climb the ladder" so that they can have a turn at exploiting; some may play a compliant and loyal role as their way of improving their lot; others may take an overtly aggressive or passive-aggressive stance. Employees will also be in conflict with their fellow employees as they compete.

In all of this jostling, clear comprehension of purpose is usually lost. We lose sight of such basics as, what is the organization's real purpose? Is it benefiting society, the environment or even its own employees? How can we bring about the true cooperative and creative effort necessary for any organization to survive and prosper? As in the wider world, there is an urgent need to find ways of living and working together in harmony.

Although better organizational structures and education can help in business, they will not cure the underlying cancer of "me first" conflict. When the pressure is on and there is no more "fat" to cushion the effects of our self-interest, each person will be looking out for him- or herself. It would be unrealistic to expect otherwise, since most businesses unabashedly appeal to and promote our greed and self-interest.

Even eminently sensible procedures like flexible working hours are all too often sabotaged by the subtle antagonisms between employers and employees. When I worked as a chartered accountant, some clients (and also some colleagues) became angry because I did not work nine-to-five and wear a three-piece suit like everyone else. They regarded this as subversive behaviour. Fortunately, I enjoyed the support of a superior who usually managed to persuade all parties to reserve their judgement until the quality of my work could speak for itself.

On the other side of the coin, I did come across several cases where employees were damaging their own best interests by using flexible working hours as paid leisure time. Whenever there is abuse, by either side, it provokes a reaction. As always, the real issue is not the particular procedure but the people executing it.

Employee participation in ownership and management is another valid concept that suffers in the execution. The antagonism between employer and employee is undoubtedly eased when the distinction between them is blurred. Unfortunately, the central problems remain. There are still those giving orders and those taking them; there is still the problem of who gets what job and how each is rewarded. In short, there is still "me first" conflict.

Procedures and structures by themselves are not enough. No matter what bargain is struck, continually changing conditions will soon make it obsolete. New technologies and new markets mean that in the future the average person will have several jobs or even different types of jobs during a career. Adaptability will be one of the most important qualities for survival, individually and collectively. Unless we can learn to resolve our fundamental conflicts, both individuals and organizations will remain locked into their respective patterns and will be unable to respond to the challenge of change.

The most profound and powerful change that can take place within the business community is personal transformation. Jobs do not really exist; people do. At all levels of collective endeavour, there needs to be some clarity and compassion; there needs to be some way of resolving conflict; there needs to be harmonious and effective action that does not originate from "me first" — that is, there needs to be non-action. These qualities can arise only within the individual. They cannot be manufactured and transplanted from the outside.

Recognition of the importance of personal transformation within the business community is just beginning. In September 1990, the Dalai Lama, the head of Tibetan Buddhism, was invited to Holland to lead a conference for top business executives. The topics were change and creativity. The chair of one of the sponsoring companies, Paul Fentener van Vlissingen, explained: "This is management development . . . in a world which changes so fast, we need managers who understand change and do not shy away from it . . . companies who are aware of changes in the world have long-term chances. If you concentrate on figures only, you will hire people who do likewise and in the end you'll get stuck."

This outlook is encouraging, but it is just the beginning of a long process. People are already mistaking the concepts of the transformational process for the thing itself. They read books or go to a seminar or a workshop for a few days, learn new concepts and techniques and come away feeling that they "know" stress reduction, change, enlightenment, love or whatever. If it were that easy, we would have reached Utopia a long time ago.

Personal transformation is necessary not only for the individual but in all relationships. It is necessary in business, government, education, the police force, the health care system and in every other aspect of society, nationally and globally. We can all see the urgent need for harmonious and constructive action. The challenge for us is to turn theory into practice. That is the ultimate "bottom line."

CONCLUSION

Many of us are experiencing confusion and suffering in our lives. In response, we quicken the pace of our lives, hoping that we can stay one step ahead of the pack in the scramble for survival and that our sheer activity will somehow fill the voids opening up all around us. There is a deepening "millennium fever," causing in some an irrational fear of extinction and in others an irrational expectation of miracles.

It is clear that if we do not find a radically different way of responding to life, if we do not change ourselves at a profound level, we court disaster. Unfortunately, experience has shown that it often takes a disaster — a famine, an earthquake, an epidemic, a massacre, a war — to arouse us to action.

Because we live in an era of accelerated change and because we have taken so much power unto ourselves, the consequences of our failure to meet life's challenges are magnified. The health of our biosphere hangs in the balance. A few more years of abuse at the current rate could very well push it over the edge. The nuclear threat has receded for the moment, but the possibility (even through accident) of the mass destruction of civilization still hangs over our heads. The magnitude of the next disaster could well make any attempts at remedial action irrelevant.

Our great material advances have backfired on the personal level as well. In the affluent West, two-income families and drudgery-saving computer advances promised shorter working hours and more leisure time. The reality has been longer working hours (as we struggle to keep up with the additional information generated), overcrowding, pollution, crime waves and a dramatic increase in debilitating and fatal stress-related diseases.

There is a feeling that "you're damned if you do and you're damned if you don't." This is because we are caught in a vicious circle of our own making. The more we bring under our control, the more there is to slip out of control; the more we attempt to solve our problems through (intellectual) analysis, the more problems we create through additional complexity.

We do not really change because, in spite of our protestations to the contrary, we do not want to change. In our present state of evolution, our actions overwhelmingly originate from our ego, that which we regard as the "I" or the "self." The primary function of the "I" is to sustain and, if possible, expand and solidify its sense of individual identity. This it does through the possession and manipulation of things, people, feelings and ideas. Real change would threaten the autocracy of the "I"; it would have to give up much of its power and control.

Individuality is exhilarating and is rightfully celebrated. In our present state of dualistic perception, however, the reverse side of individuality is usually felt as separateness. This sense of separateness is painful because we feel cut off, unfulfilled and incomplete. It is also frightening because we are mortal and vulnerable; we fear losing our individuality to outside forces (the non-I), whether these manifest as our fellow humans, God, madness, chaos or death.

All our actions may be seen as attempts to bridge the gaps of separation that we ourselves have created. We have a great need for the company of others; through sexual union we momentarily become as one with our partner. We want to move closer to God, to nature, to truth, to happiness, to security. The more we analyse and conceptualize life, however, the more fragments and gaps we create. Thus, internal is distinguished from external, mind from body, male from female, man from God, good from evil, black from white, East from West, young from old, rich from poor, now (unsatisfactory) from then (ideal). Our gap-bridging projects are endless.

We are constantly driven by beliefs and desires emanating from our "I," yet we know very little about it. We know a lot about how the "I" is related to other things (I own this, I have experienced that, I am the child of so-and-so) but almost nothing about the "I" itself. Our attention is mostly turned outward as we struggle to "rectify" our environment. Any lull in our non-stop activity is quickly filled so that we do not have to acknowledge the emptiness within.

This ignorance constitutes a fundamental blind-spot in our consciousness. It affects everything we do, whether we choose to classify it as personal, career, health, relationships, politics, economics, spirituality or otherwise. It stands to reason that we cannot find fulfilment if we do not understand what drives us, if we do not understand who we really are. Most of us do not understand because it has never occurred to us to look into ourselves to find out.

One of the most difficult but most vital things to understand is that we cannot solve our basic conflicts through systematic improvement, through so-called progress. If I see myself as separate from you, I can move closer to you, but I cannot become you. I may be clever, ruthless or "lucky" enough to amass a financial fortune and approach financial security, but I will never be secure. There will always be something more to attain, some other possible threat — the unknown, the unpredictable, death. In the dualistic scheme of things, even God has still not succeeded in defeating the Devil.

Egocentric, "me first" action is undoubtedly the cause of the division, conflict, destruction and exploitation we see and experience all the time. Religious teachers, philosophers, politicians and social commentators keep telling us so and calling for urgent change.

Our central problem is how to bring about this change. How can the "I" give up its power when its main function is to exercise power and when it is privy to every plan and scheme to deprive it of that power? Thus, even if the "I" intellectually accepts the necessity of "ego-reduction" or "ego-elimination," it quite often turns it into yet another project, yet another quest for improvement, yet another journey from now to then. The "I" is now armed with "spirituality" and exercises even greater and subtler power. It may make "progress" but will never reach its destination.

There is nothing the "I" can do but cease its activity — do nothing, surrender. Self-surrender is advocated in many religions. In Christianity, freedom from the ego comes through the "grace of God." In Buddhism, this "letting go" takes place as a result of "insight" into the essential emptiness of all phenomena. Dr. D.T. Suzuki, one of the world's greatest authorities on Zen, pointed out: "There is a strong undercurrent in Buddhist teaching to uphold the futility of all intellectual attempts in the experience of the Buddhist life, which really consists in abandoning every self-centred striving and preconceived metaphysical standpoint. This is to keep consciousness in utter purity or in a state of neutrality or blankness; in other words, to make the mind as simple as that of a child."

True self-surrender is not uncommon. When people say they have surrendered to God or to their guru, the process to which they are referring is usually not surrender but exchange. Instead of identifying with their small, personal self, they have switched their identification to a bigger, collective self. Their reward is "truth," "security" and "eternal salvation." If they had indeed attained these things, then there would be no necessity for them to defend or justify their beliefs. All too often, however, such people display strong ego reactions, albeit in the name of their saviour.

The self can surrender only by abandoning its compulsion to "do" and to "become." If it achieves this, then it simply is. It is in a state of "being." The mind is then rooted in the present and simple as a child's. "Me first" action becomes non-action or total action. It is harmonious both within and without, unfragmented by the intellect; it is free from the conditioning of the past. It can therefore totally and appropriately respond to the challenges of the moment, leaving no residue. This is the most powerful form of action possible since the present is the only reality. We worry about the future, but it never exists. Only the now exists.

As you begin to resolve and let go of conflict within yourself, wholeness, harmony, simplicity, compassion and clarity will arise in its place. These qualities will automatically manifest themselves in all aspects of your life and in all your relationships.

The new you will be the most valuable gift that you can give to the people around you and to your planet. Light is needed in all corners of our lives, and you can cast a light whether you are a firefighter, an accountant, a politician, a teacher, a doctor, a truck driver, a soldier, a businessperson, a gardener, a homemaker, a spouse or lover, a street sweeper, an artist or a priest. What matters is not the specific role you play but the quality of your underlying humanness.

One of the simplest ways to start experiencing "being" is to set aside time just to be with yourself. You need no qualifications, special skills or equipment, just a willingness to be open to and watchful of your experiences, refraining from manipulating or directing them in any manner, no matter how "reasonable" or "obvious." In time you will get to know yourself and like yourself. When that happens, you will find yourself liking everything outside yourself, because the distinctions between the two will be blurred. The Thousand-Mile Journey is completed one step at a time, and the next step is right now.

Printed in Canada